Handbook of Osteoporosis

Handbook of Osteoporosis

David M Reid
Professor of Rheumatology
Head, Division of Applied Medicine
University of Aberdeen Medical School
Aberdeen, UK

🐎 Springer Healthcare

Published by Springer Healthcare Ltd, 236 Gray's Inn Road, London, WC1X 8HB, UK.

www.springerhealthcare.com

©2011 Springer Healthcare, a part of Springer Science+Business Media.

British Library Cataloguing-in-Publication Data.

A catalogue record for this book is available from the British Library.

ISBN 978-1-907673-07-8

Although every effort has been made to ensure that drug doses and other information are presented accurately in this publication, the ultimate responsibility rests with the prescribing physician. Neither the publisher nor the authors can be held responsible for errors or for any consequences arising from the use of the information contained herein. Any product mentioned in this publication should be used in accordance with the prescribing information prepared by the manufacturers. No claims or endorsements are made for any drug or compound at present under clinical investigation.

Commissioning editor: Dinah Alam
Project editor: Alison Whitehouse
Designer: Joe Harvey
Artworker: Sissan Mollerfors
Production: Marina Maher

Contents

Author biographies   vii

1   Introduction   **1**
   Epidemiology of osteoporosis   1
   Prevalence of osteoporosis in postmenopausal women?   2
   Risk factors for postmenopausal osteopaenia and osteoporosis   2
   Clinical features of osteoporosis   4
   Quality-of-life issues in women with postmenopausal osteoporosis 10

2   Pathophysiology   **13**
   Normal bone remodelling cycle   13
   Inhibitors and stimulators of bone remodelling   16
   Age-related changes in bone mineral density   16
   Role of oestrogen in bone remodelling   19

3   Prevention   **23**
   Population strategies   23
   Targeted approaches   27

4   Investigation and diagnosis   **33**
   Definition and diagnostic criteria   33
   Assessment of osteoporosis   35
   The gold standard for diagnosis   45

5   Fracture risk assessment   **49**
   BMD and fracture risk   49
   Limitations of BMD   52
   Biochemical markers of bone turnover   52
   Biochemical markers and fracture risk   53
   Biochemical markers and treatment response   56
   WHO fracture Risk Assessment Tool (FRAX)   57

6   Non-pharmacological and adjunctive management   61

Non-pharmacological approaches to postmenopausal osteoporosis   61

Goals of intervention   61

Diet and nutrition   62

Exercise   70

Smoking cessation   72

Alcohol consumption   72

Prevention of and protection against falls   72

7   Pharmacological treatment   77

Bisphosphonates   78

Oestrogen   93

Calcitonin   99

Calcium plus vitamin D   101

Parathyroid hormone derivatives   102

Strontium ranelate   105

Denosumab   107

Guidelines for treatment of postmenopausal osteoporosis   110

Current thinking about combination therapy   111

8   Long-term management   117

Pain management   117

Compliance   119

Author biography

David M Reid, MD, FRCPEdin, FRCPLon, holds a Personal Chair of Rheumatology at the University of Aberdeen, Scotland, UK. He is Head of the Division of Applied Medicine at the University of Aberdeen. He graduated in 1975 from the University of Aberdeen and after academic training at the University of Edinburgh returned to Aberdeen in 1983.

He has published over 200 original papers and reviews, largely on his current research interests which include the utility of bone mass assessment, assessment of risk of fracture, secondary osteoporosis and the assessment of long-term disease activity and drug adverse effects in rheumatic diseases.

He is the current chairman of the Board of Trustees of the National Osteoporosis Society (NOS) and has recently taken the lead in the NOS-endorsed guidelines on breast cancer treatment induced bone loss management.

Author biography

Chapter 1

Introduction

Epidemiology of osteoporosis

Osteoporosis is defined as a skeletal disorder characterized by compromised bone strength predisposing a person to an increased risk of fracture, bone strength reflecting the integration of bone density and bone quality [1]. Osteoporosis affects an estimated 75 million people in Europe, Japan and the USA [2]. Its prevalence increases with age, and it mainly affects postmenopausal women and older men. After accounting for age, the risk of fracture for postmenopausal women is about three times that for men, partly because women have a lower peak bone mass and partly because of hormonal changes that occur at the menopause. The lifetime risk of osteoporotic fracture in a 50-year-old woman is 40%, similar to that for coronary heart disease (Figure 1.1) [2].

In 1990 there were 1.7 million hip fractures worldwide. With the anticipated increases in world population and life expectancy, this figure

Estimated lifetime risk of fracture in Caucasian men and women at age 50		
	Lifetime risk of fracture (%) (95% CI)	
Fracture site	Women	Men
Proximal femur	17.5 (16.8–18.2)	6.0 (5.6–6.5)
Vertebra*	15.6 (14.8–16.3)	5.0 (4.6–5.4)
Distal forearm	16.0 (15.7–16.7)	2.5 (2.2–3.1)
Any of the above	39.7 (38.7–40.6)	13.1 (12.4–13.7)

*Clinically diagnosed fractures

Figure 1.1 Estimated lifetime risk of fracture in Caucasian men and women at age 50.
CI, confidence interval. Reproduced with permission from World Health Organization (WHO). Assessment of Fracture Risk and its Application to Screening for Postmenopausal Osteoporosis. WHO Technical Report Series 843. Geneva: WHO, 1994.

is predicted to rise to 6.3 million by 2050 (Figure 1.2) [2]. Accordingly, the World Health Organization has identified osteoporosis as a priority health issue and called for a global strategy for the prevention and control of the disease.

Compared with Caucasians, blacks have about one-third and Asians and Hispanics about half the risk of hip fracture. Currently, the majority of hip fractures occur in Europe and North America. However, demographic shifts over the next 50 years will lead to huge increases in the numbers of elderly people in Africa, Asia and South America. Consequently, the burden of the disease will shift from the developed to the developing countries (Figure 1.3). By 2050, 75% of the estimated, expected 6.3 million hip fractures will occur in the developing countries [2].

Prevalence of osteoporosis in postmenopausal women

Around 85% of all osteoporotic fractures occur in women. In Europe, more than one-third of women aged 50 years or older are believed to have osteoporosis, according to the World Health Organization diagnostic criteria [2,4]. The prevalence varies widely according to nationality and ethnicity, however. The disease is most common in Scandinavia, New Zealand, and the United States, intermediate in Britain, Southern Europe, and Asia, and least common in South Africa [2].

The assessment and diagnosis of osteoporosis is discussed in more detail in Chapter 4.

Risk factors for postmenopausal osteopaenia and osteoporosis

Osteoporosis occurs primarily as a result of normal ageing. In addition to age, the major risk factors for osteoporosis are menopausal status, genetics, and lifestyle. The risk factors for postmenopausal osteopaenia and osteoporosis are summarized in Figure 1.4.

Secondary causes of bone loss including certain medical conditions (Figure 1.5) and medications (Figure 1.6). Osteoporosis that develops secondary to other pathologies or the use of certain medications is not

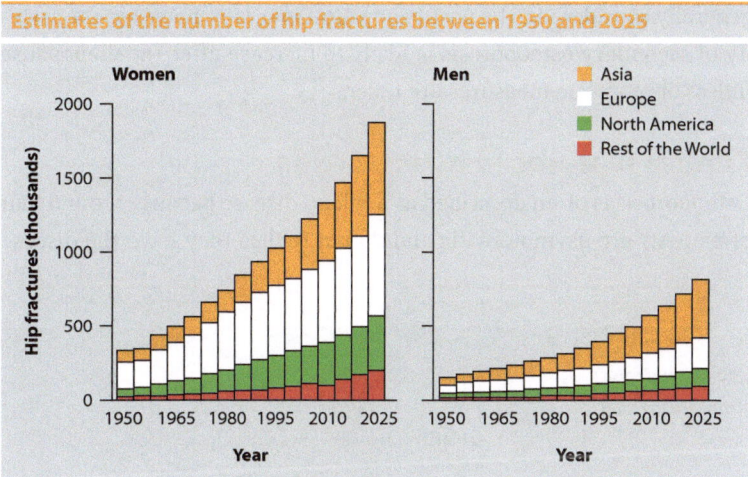

Figure 1.2 Estimates of the number of hip fractures between 1950 and 2025. Reproduced with permission from World Health Organization (WHO). Prevention and Management of Osteoporosis. Report of a WHO Scientific Group. WHO Technical Report Series 921. Geneva: WHO, 2003.

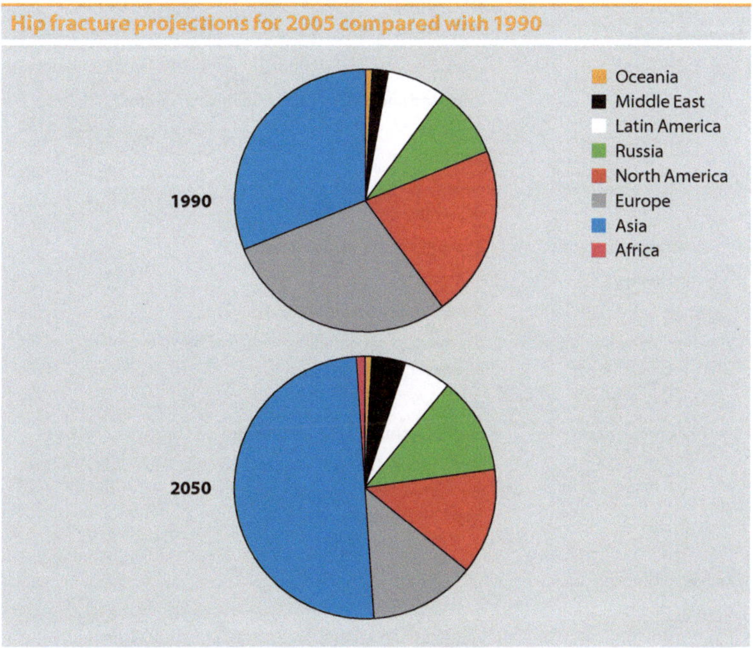

Hip fracture projections for 2005 compared with 1990

Figure 1.3 Hip fracture projections for 2005 compared with 1990. Data from aCooper et al. [3].

generally considered to be postmenopausal in origin; however, the severity of secondary osteoporosis is likely to increase after the menopause unless appropriate measures are taken.

Clinical features of osteoporosis

Osteoporosis is often described as a 'silent' disease because around half of patients are asymptomatic and do not realise they have the disease

Risk factors for postmenopausal osteopaenia and osteoporosis	
Risk factors	**Comments**
Modifiable factors	
Cigarette smoking	–
Immobility	Sedentary lifestyle or history of long-term bed rest/immobility
Excessive alcohol intake	–
Poor diet	Insufficient fruit and vegetables
Vitamin D Deficiency	Vitamin D is required for optimal calcium absorbtion
Protein/energy malnutrition	Low calcium intake, e.g. low intake of dairy products and high intake of low-calcium carbonated soft drinks
Unmodifiable factors	
Age	Protein/energy malnutrition
	Increased age is associated with decreased BMD
	Bone loss is most rapid in the years immediately following menopause
Caucasian or Asian race	Genetic factors are almost certainly the reason for racial differences in BMD
Family history of osteoporosis	Especially a first-degree relative
Early menopause	> 45 years
	Natural or surgically induced
Cessation of menstruation before menopause	e.g. because of conditions such as anorexia or bulimia, or excessive exercise
Previous low-impact fracture	–
Low peak bone mass	Peak bone mass is 60–80% determined by genetic factors
	Other influential factors include lifestyle (including exercise levels), hormones (e.g. growth hormone) and nutrition (calcium and protein intake)
Elevated bone turnover	–
Bone quality and architecture	–
Low BMI	–
Nulliparity	Increased parity is associated with increased BMD

Figure 1.4 Risk factors for postmenopausal osteopaenia and osteoporosis.

until they suffer a fracture. Furthermore, only one-third of osteoporosis-related fractures come to medical attention (Figure 1.7). Undetected fractures may lead to chronic pain, disability and deformity. Other than in clinically recognized fractures, osteoporosis may be suspected in the presence of kyphosis and loss of height.

Diseases and disorders associated with an increased risk of osteoporosis
Endocrine
Thyrotoxicosis
Hyperparathyroidism
Cushing syndrome
Insulin-dependent diabetes mellitus
Addison disease
Ectopic adrenocorticotropic hormone syndrome
Gastrointestinal
Severe liver disease – especially primary biliary cirrhosis
Gastrectomy
Malabsorption syndromes including coeliac disease
Metabolic and nutritional
Haemophilia
Hypophosphatasia
Congenital erythrocytic porphyria
Chronic renal disease
Idiopathic hypercalciuria
Haemochromatosis
Osteogenesis imperfecta
Mastocytosis
Amyloidosis
Thalassaemia and chronic haemolytic disease
Parenteral nutrition
Neoplasia
Myelomatosis
Tumour secretion of parathyroid hormone-related peptide
Lymphoma and leukaemia
Other
Chronic obstructive pulmonary disease
Epidermolysis bullosa
Pregnancy

Figure 1.5 Diseases and disorders associated with an increased risk of osteoporosis.
Data from World Health Organization [2].

Any bone can fracture as a result of osteoporosis but the hip, spine and wrist are most susceptible. Osteoporotic fractures are often caused by low-impact trauma, such as a fall from standing. However people with osteoporosis are also more likely to have a fracture following high-energy impact than are their normal counterparts.

The incidence, morbidity, and mortality associated with the three most common osteoporotic fractures are illustrated in Figures 1.8, 1.9 and 1.10.

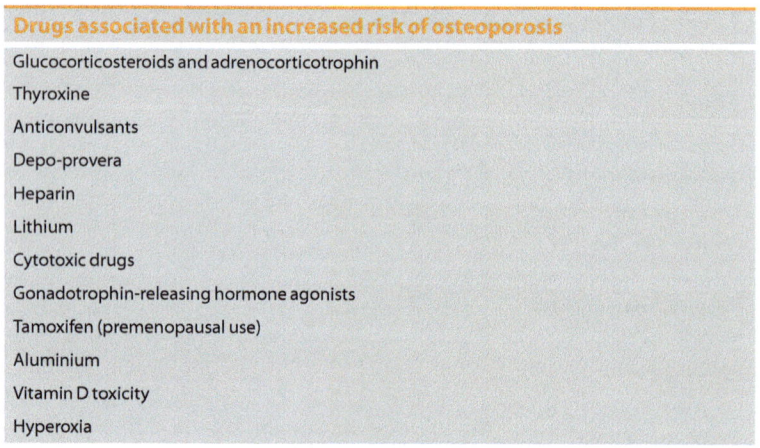

Drugs associated with an increased risk of osteoporosis

Glucocorticosteroids and adrenocorticotrophin

Thyroxine

Anticonvulsants

Depo-provera

Heparin

Lithium

Cytotoxic drugs

Gonadotrophin-releasing hormone agonists

Tamoxifen (premenopausal use)

Aluminium

Vitamin D toxicity

Hyperoxia

Figure 1.6 Drugs associated with an increased risk of osteoporosis.

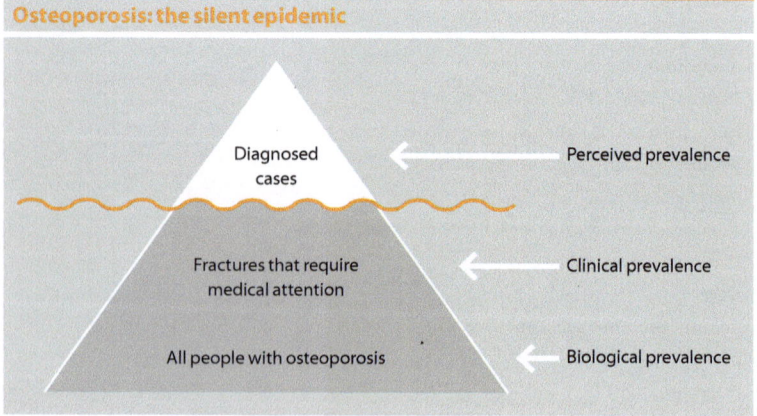

Osteoporosis: the silent epidemic

Diagnosed cases — Perceived prevalence

Fractures that require medical attention — Clinical prevalence

All people with osteoporosis — Biological prevalence

Figure 1.7 Osteoporosis: the silent epidemic.

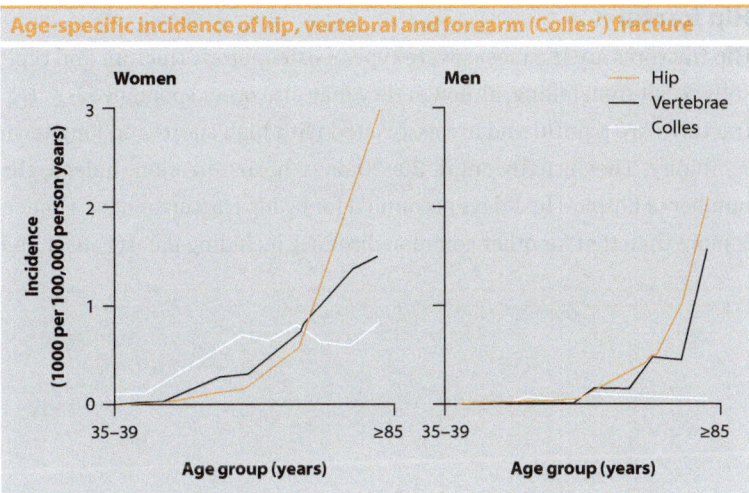

Figure 1.8 Age-specific incidence of hip, vertebral and forearm (Colles') fracture. Data from Cooper and Melton LJ III [5].

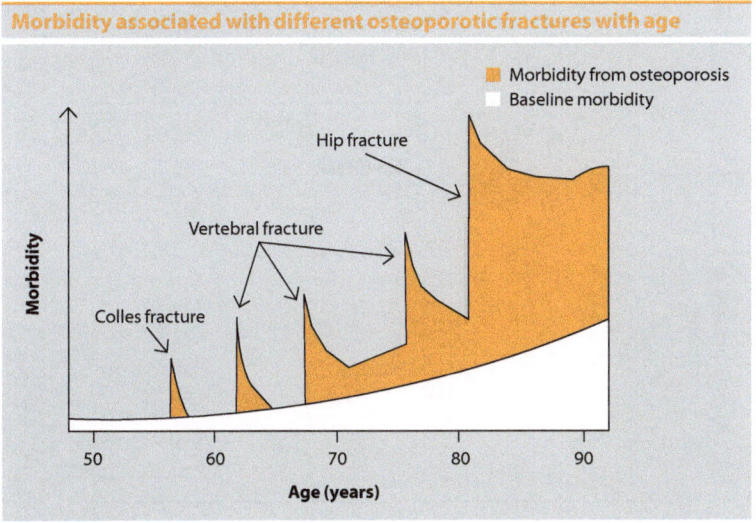

Figure 1.9 Morbidity associated with different osteoporotic fractures with age. Colles' fracture commonly occurs in women in their mid-50s and has short-term sequelae. Repeated vertebral fractures occurring at a later age may give rise to permanent morbidity. Hip fractures occur at an average age of 80 years in developed countries and usually result in permanent morbidity. Reproduced with permission from Kanis JA, Johnell O. The burden of osteoporosis. J Endocrinol Invest 1999;22:583–588.

Hip fracture

Hip fractures are the most severe type of osteoporotic fracture and typically result from falling, although they may also occur spontaneously. Hip fractures are painful and are associated with high short- and long-term morbidity. They usually entail 20–30 days' hospitalization. Indeed, the number of hospital bed-days accounted for by hip fracture among women is more than that for other common diseases, including breast cancer and

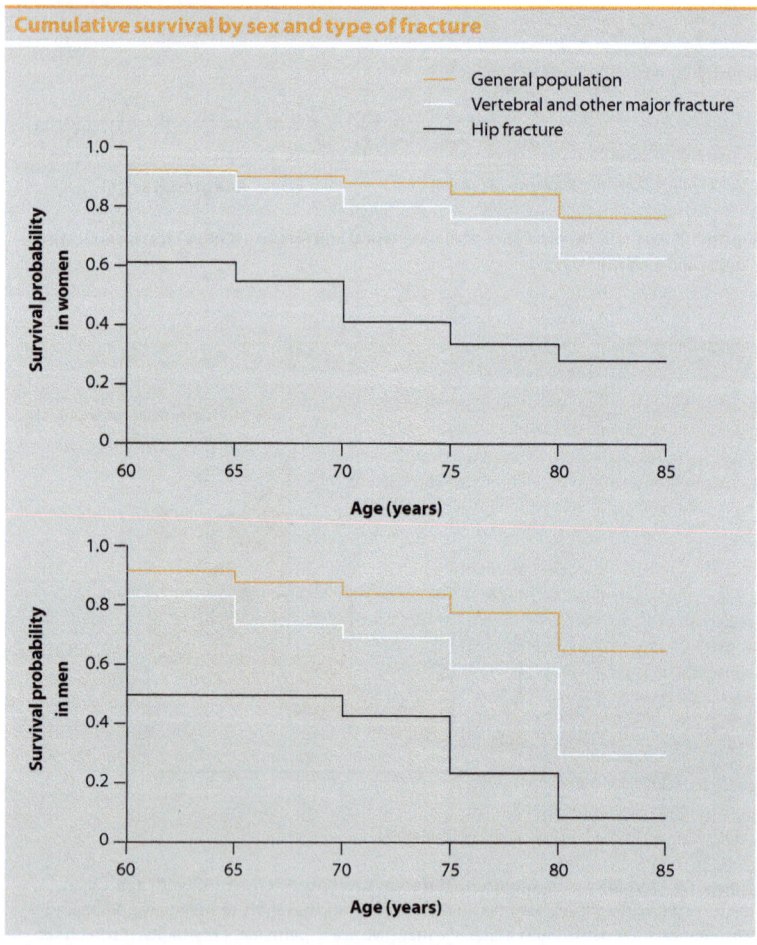

Figure 1.10 Cumulative survival by sex and type of fracture. Reproduced with permission from Center JR, Nguyen TV, Schneider D et al. Mortality after all major types of osteoporotic fracture in men and women: an observational study. Lancet 1999; 353:878–882.

coronary heart disease (Figure 1.11) [6]. Recovery from hip fracture is often complicated by prolonged immobility, and half of the patients suffer long-term morbidity. Following a hip fracture, 25% of patients require long-term nursing home care and 15–30% will die in the first year [2].

Vertebral fracture

Vertebral compression fractures are the most frequent type of osteoporotic fracture and occur spontaneously or as a result of lifting or other minimal trauma. Typical symptoms include back pain, progressive loss of height, and kyphosis. Many vertebral fractures are asymptomatic or cause too few clinical symptoms to provoke clinical investigation, and they rarely lead to hospitalization. Nevertheless vertebral fractures are associated with increased mortality and a significant decrease in the quality of life, particularly in psychosocial domains.

Forearm fracture

Fractures of the forearm are usually caused by falling on an outstretched hand, and more than 80% occur at the distal radius (Colles' fracture). Although they cause less morbidity than hip or vertebral fractures, forearm

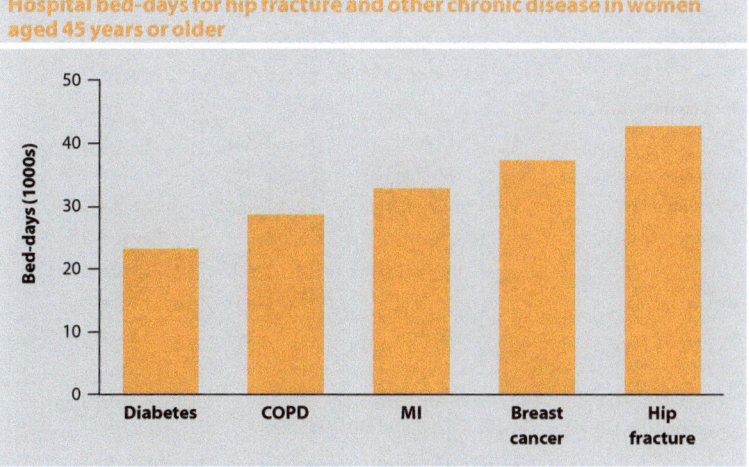

Figure 1.11 Hospital bed-days for hip fracture and other chronic disease in women aged 45 years or older. COPD, chronic obstructive pulmonary disease; MI, myocardial infarction. Data from Kanis et al. [6].

fractures are painful and usually require manipulation or even surgery to reposition the bones, followed by 4–6 weeks in plaster. Complications such as algodystrophy are common and half of patients report fair or poor functional outcomes at 6 months [2].

Quality-of-life issues in women with postmenopausal osteoporosis

Osteoporosis per se does not result in overall loss of health-related quality of life. Rather, the disease burden in osteoporosis reflects the increased risk of fracture and the associated morbidity and mortality. While the detrimental impact of hip fractures on quality of life has long been known, the burden associated with vertebral fractures has only recently been recognized. Furthermore, all common osteoporotic fractures interfere with activities of daily living, albeit to different degrees (Figure 1.12).

Influence of common osteoporotic fractures on activities of daily living			
Physical or functional impairment	**Odds of impairment (95% CI)***		
	Hip fracture	**Spine fracture**	**Wrist fracture**
Activities			
Cook meals	11.1 (2.4–51.7)	6.9 (1.6–31.0)	10.2 (3.3–31.9)
Heavy housework	2.8 (1.0–7.9)	2.1 (0.8–5.6)	1.6 (0.9–2.9)
Put socks on	1.6 (0.6–4.4)	1.7 (0.6–4.6)	1.1 (0.5–2.2)
Shop	4.6 (1.4–15.7)	5.2 (1.6–16.8)	3.3 (1.3–8.0)
Movements			
Bend	2.7 (1.1–6.8)	3.1 (1.2–7.8)	1.2 (0.6–2.5)
Climb stairs	2.6 (1.0–7.0)	2.2 (0.7–6.7)	1.8 (0.9–3.7)
Descend stairs	4.1 (1.5–11.1)	4.2 (1.5–11.6)	2.5 (1.2–5.3)
Get into/out of car	1.3 (0.5–3.5)	2.1 (0.8–5.6)	1.3 (0.6–2.5)
Lift	1.1 (0.3–3.6)	3.4 (1.2–9.5)	1.3 (0.6–2.6)
Reach	1.5 (0.5–4.5)	0.7 (0.2–3.1)	1.8 (0.9–3.7)
Walk	3.6 (1.4–9.0)	2.7 (1.0–7.4)	1.6 (0.8–3.4)

* Likelihood of the impairment following fracture, after adjusting for age, body mass index, oestrogen use, visual impairment and reduced mental status.

Figure 1.12 Influence of common osteoporotic fractures on activities of daily living. CI, confidence interval. Data from Greendale GA, Barrett-Connor E, Ingles S, et al. Latae physical and functional effects of osteoporotic fracture in women: the Rancho Bernardo Study. J Am Geriatr Soc 1995;43:955-61.

Osteoporotic fractures can have negative physical, psychological, economic and social consequences, all of which have the potential to diminish women's quality of life. Moreover, a single fracture increases the risk for subsequent fractures, leading to a 'downward spiral' of worsening health-related quality of life. These consequences are summarized in Figure 1.13.

References

1   NIH Consensus Development Panel on Osteoporosis Prevention, Diagnosis, and Therapy. Consensus panel on osteoporosis prevention. 2001. JAMA 2001; 285:785–95.
2   World Health Organization (WHO). Prevention and management of osteoporosis. report of a WHO scientific group. WHO Technical Report Series 921. Geneva: WHO, 2003.
3   Cooper C, Campion G, Melton LJ III. Hip fractures in the elderly: a world-wide projection. Osteoporos Int. 1992;2:285–9.
4   World Health Organization (WHO). Assessment of fracture risk and its application to screening for postmenopausal osteoporosis. WHO Technical Report Series 843. Geneva: WHO, 1994.
5   Cooper C, Melton LJ III. Epidemiology of osteoporosis. Trends Endocrinol Metab 1992;3:224–229.
6   Kanis JA, Delmas P, Burckhardt P, et al. Guidelines for diagnosis and management of osteoporosis. The European Foundation for Osteoporosis and Bone Disease. Osteoporos Int 1997;7:390–406.

Negative consequences of osteoporotic fractures
Physical
Pain (acute/chronic)
Fatigue
Deformity/disability
Functional impairment
Prolonged immobility
Complications (e.g. algodystrophy)
Psychological
Depression
Anxiety (especially fear of falling)
Loss of self-esteem
Perceived poor global health status
Economic
Inpatient care
Nursing home care
Outpatient care
Social
Isolation
Loss of independence
Loss of social roles

Figure 1.13 Negative consequences of osteoporotic fractures.

Chapter 2

Pathophysiology

Normal bone remodelling cycle

Bone structure and composition

Bone is a dynamic living tissue composed of metabolically active cells integrated into a rigid framework. The main constituents of bone are an organic matrix and a complex crystalline salt. The combination of soft collagen overlaid with hard mineral creates a structure that is flexible yet resilient to stress.

The adult skeleton contains two types of bone: cortical (compact) and trabecular (spongy or cancellous) bone. Cortical bone makes up the dense outer shell of the bone and constitutes around 80% of the human skeleton. It is found mainly at the end of long bones and the inner part of flat bones, and it consists of bone cells arranged concentrically around central canals (Haversian systems) that contain blood and lymphatic vessels, nerves and connective tissue.

The remaining 20% of the skeleton is trabecular bone, which forms the inner layer of the bone and has a honeycomb-like structure. Trabecular bone makes up most of the vertebral bodies and the ends of the long bones, known as epiphysis. It has a greater surface area than cortical bone and is remodelled more rapidly. Trabecular bone is also more rapidly affected by conditions associated with increased bone turnover than cortical bone, and is, therefore, susceptible to bone loss.

The structure of bone is shown in Figure 2.1.

Bone remodelling

Bone is in a state of flux throughout life. Bone cells undergo continuous modelling and/or remodelling to allow the skeleton to grow and adapt to prevailing needs.

Modelling is the process by which new bone is formed, permitting the shape and strength of the skeleton to be altered. This occurs primarily during childhood.

Remodelling, by contrast, is the process responsible for bone maintenance and repair. It is the predominant process in the adult and consists of gradual, controlled bone destruction and formation (Figure 2.2). Remodelling allows the bone architecture to be altered in response to factors such as mechanical loading, but without changing the overall skeletal size. In the adult skeleton, 5–10% of bone is remodelled every year. Remodelling does not occur uniformly throughout the skeleton but at discrete sites; 80% of remodelling occurs in trabecular bone.

Bone anatomy and microanatomy

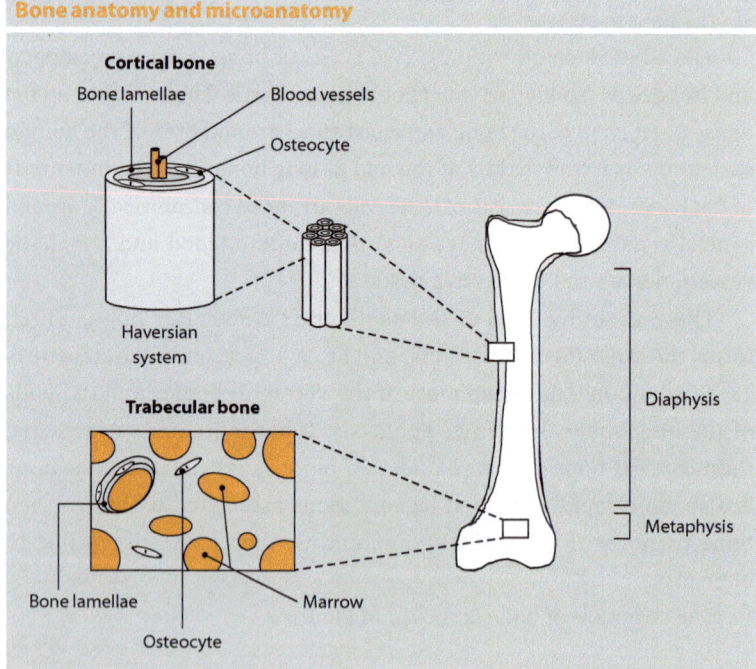

Figure 2.1 Bone anatomy and microanatomy.

Bone cells

Bone turnover involves at least three distinct cell types (Figure 2.3):

- **osteoblasts** are mononuclear cells that synthesize new bone matrix and help regulate mineralization;
- **osteocytes** are mature cells involved in mineral recycling and stress detection; and
- **osteoclasts** are multinucleated giant bone-resorbing cells.

The functions of osteoclasts and osteoblasts are closely linked, with osteoclastic bone resorption being followed by an increase in osteoblastic bone formation. The production of new bone matrix, and its subsequent calcification, is known as osteogenesis. The dissolution of bone mineral and organic substrates is known as resorption or osteolysis, the latter term usually used as part of a pathological process.

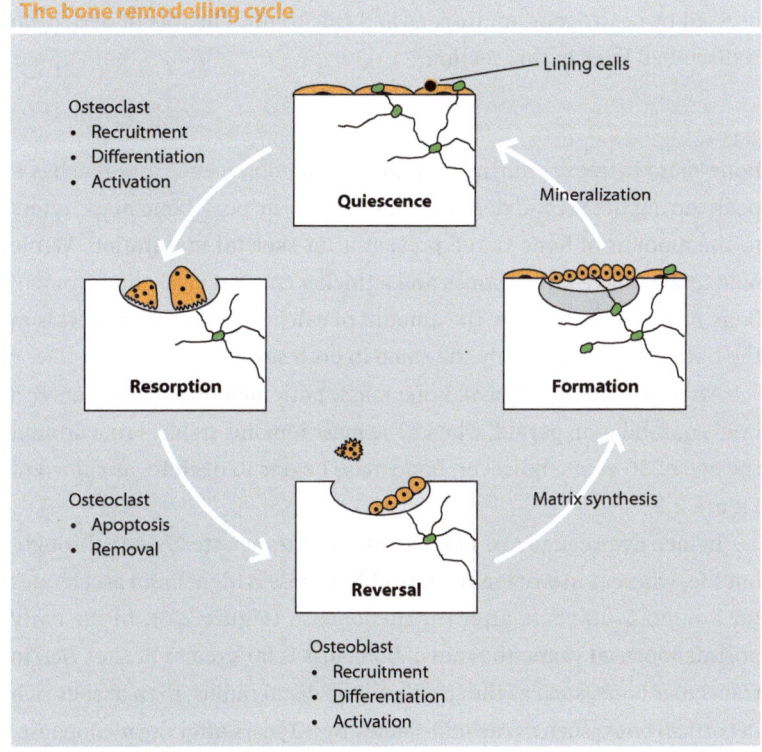

The bone remodelling cycle

Lining cells

Osteoclast
- Recruitment
- Differentiation
- Activation

Quiescence

Mineralization

Resorption

Formation

Osteoclast
- Apoptosis
- Removal

Matrix synthesis

Reversal

Osteoblast
- Recruitment
- Differentiation
- Activation

Figure 2.2 The bone remodelling cycle.

Inhibitors and stimulators of bone remodelling

Bone remodelling is a highly complex process that is regulated by systemic and locally produced growth factors, cytokines, and hormones. Some of the main stimulators and inhibitors of bone remodelling are shown in Figure 2.4.

Mechanical stimuli and areas of microdamage are likely to be important in determining the sites at which remodelling occurs in the normal skeleton. Increased bone remodelling may result from the local or systemic release of inflammatory cytokines, such as interleukin-1 and tumour necrosis factor. Calciotropic hormones such as parathyroid hormone and vitamin D act together to increase bone remodelling on a systemic basis, allowing skeletal calcium to be mobilized for maintenance of plasma calcium homeostasis. Bone remodelling is also increased by other hormones, such as thyroid hormone and growth hormone, and is suppressed by oestrogens, androgens and calcitonin. The role of oestrogen is discussed later in this section.

Age-related changes in bone mineral density

Bone mass increases during childhood and adolescence and reaches a peak during the second decade of life. The term 'peak bone mass' refers to the amount of bone tissue present after skeletal maturation. While men tend to have larger bones and a thicker cortical layer than women, bone mineral density (i.e. the amount of calcium and other minerals in the bone) is approximately the same in both sexes.

After attainment of peak bone mass, both men and women enter a brief consolidation period, when bone mass remains stable. From around the age of 30 years, however, bone mass begins to decline, as shown in Figure 2.5.

In men age-related loss of bone mass occurs at a steady rate throughout life, whereas in women the rate of bone loss is higher and accelerates for around 5–10 years after the menopause (Figure 2.6). In the early postmenopausal years, the rate of bone loss is far greater at sites rich in trabecular bone, such as the spine and the distal radius, than at sites rich in cortical bone, such as the mid-radius. By 20 years after the menopause, bone loss is still greater at trabecular sites but the difference is smaller.

Cells involved in bone remodelling

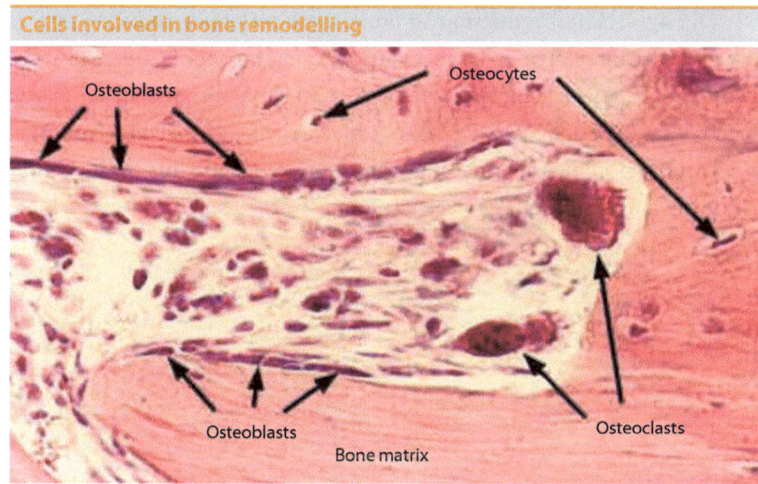

Figure 2.3 Cells involved in bone remodelling. Originally published in Rizzoli R, Atlas of Postmenopausal Osteoporosis, 2nd edition, London: Current Medicine Group Limited, 2005, by courtesy of David King, Department of Anatomy, Southern Illinois University School of Medicine, Carbondale, Illinois, USA.

Modulators of bone remodelling

Stimulators	
Systemic hormones	**Locally acting factors**
Parathyroid hormone	Interleukin-1
1,25-dihydroxyvitamin D	Tumour necrosis factor
Parathyroid hormone-related protein	Insulin-like growth factor
Growth hormone	Interleukin-6
Thyroid hormone	Receptor activated nuclear factor kappa B ligand
	Prostaglandins
	Macrophage-colony stimulating factor
Inhibitors	
Systemic hormones	**Locally acting factors**
Oestrogens	Osteoprotegerin
Androgens	Mechanical loading*
Progesterone	Interferon gamma
Calcitonin	Interleukin-4, -10, -13, and -18
	Transforming growth factor beta

*Inhibits bone resorption, but stimulates formation

Figure 2.4 Modulators of bone remodelling. Reproduced with permission from Rizzoli R. Atlas of Postmenopausal Osteoporosis, 2nd edition. London: Current Medicine Group Limited, 2005.

The age-related reduction in bone mass reflects a reduced rate of bone formation relative to bone resorption; in other words, the resorptive activity of osteoclasts increases relative to the bone-producing activity of osteoblasts. As bone mass decreases, the cortical layer becomes progressively thinner while the inner layer becomes less dense due to trabecular thinning and loss of connectivity (Figure 2.7).

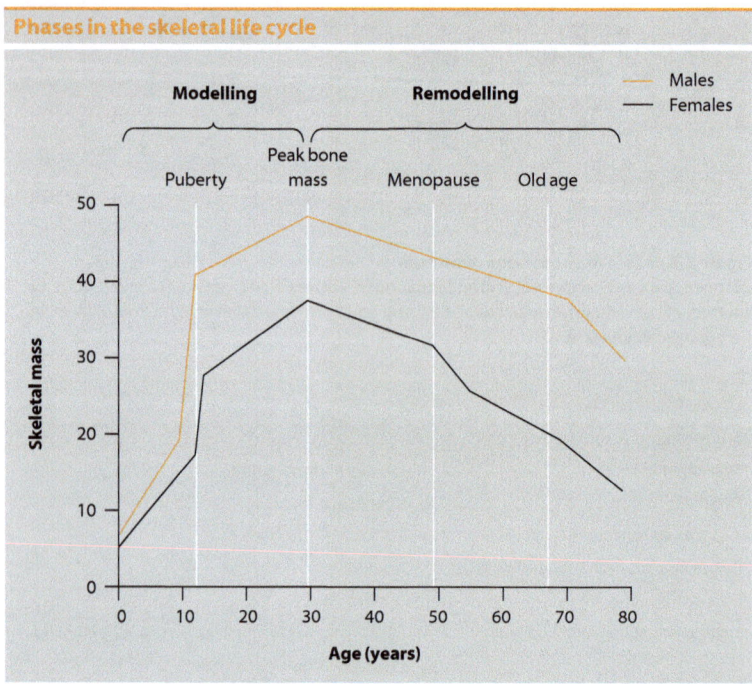

Phases in the skeletal life cycle

Figure 2.5 **Phases in the skeletal life cycle.**

Normal rate of bone loss in men and women over 30 years of age

		Bone loss (% per year)
Women	Postmenopause:	
	> 10 years	1
	> 5–10 years	2–3
	Premenopause*	1
Men		0.3–0.5

*Some authors suggest bone loss is lower, at 0.3–0.6%, in this group

Figure 2.6 **Normal rate of bone loss in men and women over 30 years of age.** Data from Kanis [1]

Peak bone mass is a major determinant of the risk of osteoporotic fracture and is governed by a number of factors, including heredity, sex, diet and nutrition, hormonal status, weight-bearing physical activity, and exposure to risk factors (Figure 2.8). Genetic factors are thought to be most important, accounting for 60–80% of the observed variance in adult bone mass.

Role of oestrogen in bone remodelling

Oestrogen has two key roles in bone health. First, the hormone is essential for normal bone maturation and mineral acquisition, i.e. the achievement of peak bone mass. Second, oestrogen maintains bone mass in adult life through its regulation of bone remodelling. As described below, oestrogen deficiency leads to a reduction in bone mass as well as deterioration in the bone microarchitecture – the two hallmarks of osteoporosis. Oestrogen deficiency is therefore a major determinant of age-related bone loss and a leading cause of osteoporosis in both women and men [2].

Oestrogen deficiency can cause loss of bone through direct action on bone cells that are involved in restraining bone turnover, and through the loss of action of oestrogen on the intestine and kidney, which regulate

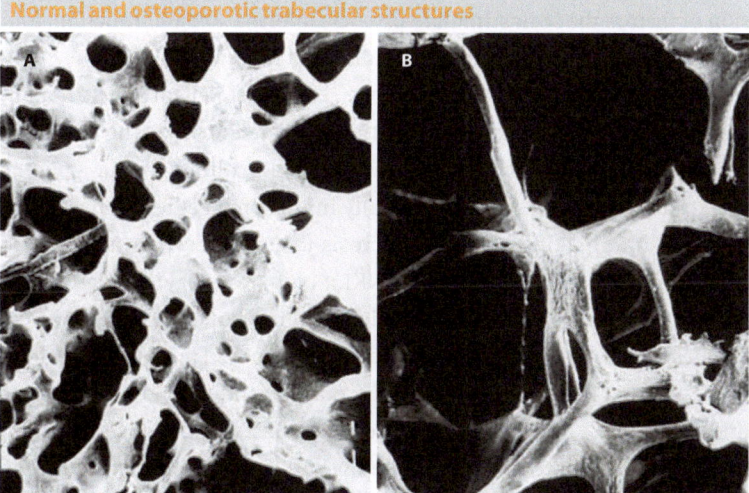

Normal and osteoporotic trabecular structures

Figure 2.7 Normal and osteoporotic trabecular structures. Reproduced with kind permission from Kosek J, Stanford University School of Medicine, Stanford, California, USA.

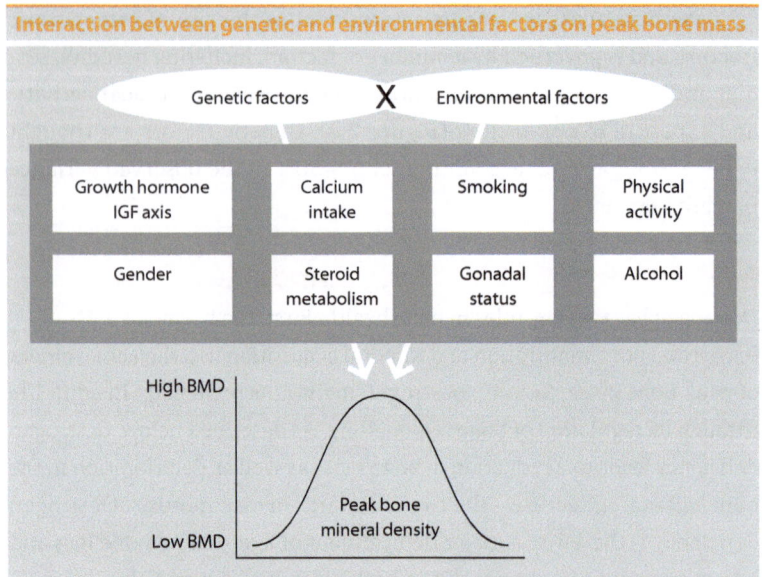

Figure 2.8 Interaction between genetic and environmental factors on peak bone mass.
Reproduced with permission from Rizzoli R. Atlas of Postmenopausal Osteoporosis, 2nd edition. London: Current Medicine Group Limited, 2005.

extraskeletal calcium levels. Oestrogen can also modulate the expression of factors that can stimulate osteoclast formation and function, and induce osteoclast apoptosis, as summarized in Figure 2.9.

The mechanisms by which oestrogen exerts its skeletal effects remain to be clearly defined. Many of its actions are mediated via the two main oestrogen receptor (ER) subtypes, ERα and ERβ, although non-genomic effects also occur. Oestrogen normally inhibits molecules such as interleukin-1, interleukin-6, tumour necrosis factor-α, receptor activator of nuclear factor kappa B ligand (RANKL), and granulocyte–macrophage colony-stimulating factor, all of which enhance bone resorption [2].

Oestrogen deficiency therefore leads to increased production of these proresorptive factors, resulting in increased production of osteoblasts and osteoclasts, increased lifespan of osteoclasts, and reduced lifespan of osteoblasts and osteocytes. The overall result is accelerated bone turnover and an imbalance between resorption and formation, leading to loss of bone tissue [3].

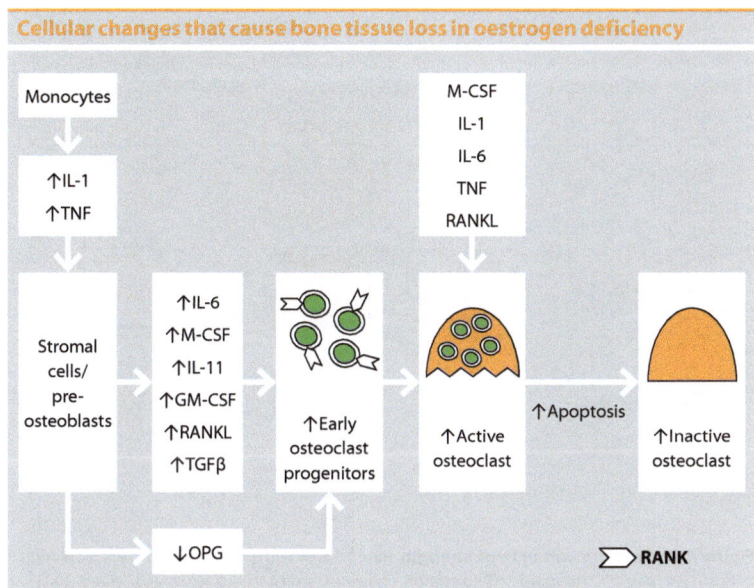

Figure 2.9 Cellular changes that cause bone tissue loss in oestrogen deficiency. Reproduced with permission from Rizzoli R. Atlas of Postmenopausal Osteoporosis, 2nd edition. London: Current Medicine Group Limited, 2005.

Oestrogen deficiency also contributes to a deterioration in the microarchitecture of bone and a reduction in bone strength. As shown in Figure 2.10, bone strength is determined by bone geometry, cortical thickness, porosity, trabecular bone morphology, and intrinsic properties of bony tissue. Bone remodelling results in modification of major determinants of bone strength, such as mass, microarchitecture (trabecular volume, connectivity, and thickness), geometry (outer diameter, and cortical thickness), and factors related to the intrinsic mechanical quality of bony tissue (mineralization, collagen fibril orientation and links, porosity, and microdamage).

References

1   Kanis JA. Osteoporosis. Oxford: Blackwell Science; 1997.
2   World Health Organization (WHO). Prevention and management of osteoporosis. report of a WHO scientific group. WHO Technical Report Series 921. Geneva: WHO, 2003.
3   Hofbauer LC, Schoppet M. Clinical implications of the osteoprotegerin/RANKL/RANK system for bone and vascular diseases. JAMA 2004;292:490–5.

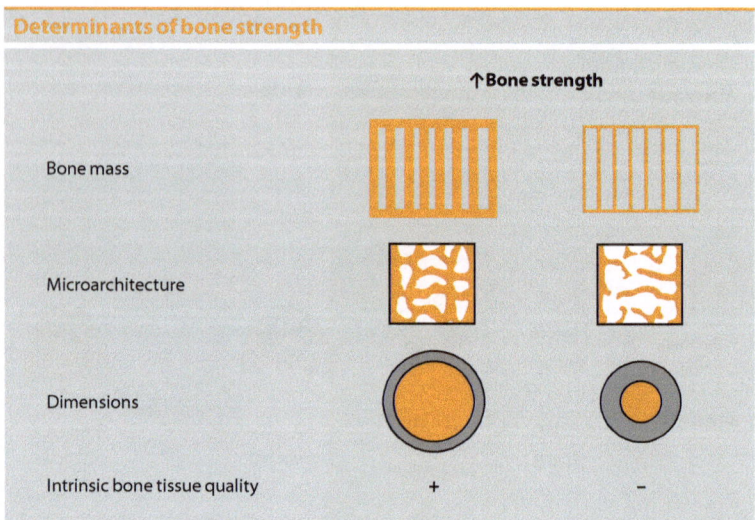

Figure 2.10 Determinants of bone strength. Reproduced with permission from Rizzoli R. Atlas of Postmenopausal Osteoporosis, 2nd edition. London: Current Medicine Group Limited, 2005.

Chapter 3

Prevention

The prevention of osteoporosis includes both population-based and targeted approaches (Figure 3.1). The goal of population-based strategies is to reduce the risk of osteoporotic fracture and the ensuing clinical and economic burden. Possible population-level approaches include lifestyle/behavioural changes and/or a mass screening programme. Targeted strategies, on the other hand, attempt to identify people at high risk of osteoporosis as indicated by the presence of risk factors, including a prior fragility fracture, and to assess and treat as appropriate.

In most areas, primary care practitioners and primary care teams are in the best position to be able to identify and treat at-risk patients. The number likely to be at highest risk within an average practice is small enough to be manageable (Figure 3.2), yet tackling this group can have a dramatic impact on future fracture rates.

Population strategies
Lifestyle and behavioural changes

Bone strength in later life, when fracture risk is highest, is determined by three factors: the accrual of skeletal mass during childhood and adolescence, the extent to which peak bone mass is maintained during young adulthood, and the amount of bone lost in later life. The three processes differ, as does the role of various lifestyle interventions in each period. Thus, interventions aimed at children may differ from those directed at adults, although some are relevant at all ages.

The main non-pharmacological interventions are dietary (particularly calcium and vitamin D intake), exercise (as an anabolic stimulus and to optimize skeletal load-bearing efficiency), the maintenance of body weight, and the avoidance of skeletal insults (e.g. smoking, high alcohol intake or exogenous glucocorticoid). For postmenopausal women, there is convincing evidence for a slowing of the rate of bone loss with regular physical exercise and sufficient intake of vitamin D and calcium, and for an increase in the risk of bone loss with high consumption of alcohol (>3–4 units per day), smoking and low body weight. The timing of puberty and levels of sex hormones during adulthood could also be importatnt. Recommended preventive strategies for patients therefore include:

- ensure sufficient dietary calcium and vitamin D intake (with supplements if necessary),
- take regular weight-bearing and resistance exercise,
- limit alcohol intake to less than 3–4 units per day and
- maintain a healthy body weight.

Practical strategies for preventing osteoporosis

Population strategies

- Population-wide improvement of bone mineral density
- Population screening

Targeted strategies (selective case finding)

- 'Opportunistically' identify individuals at high risk
- 'Search and rescue' strategies for high-risk groups

Figure 3.1 Practical strategies for preventing osteoporosis.

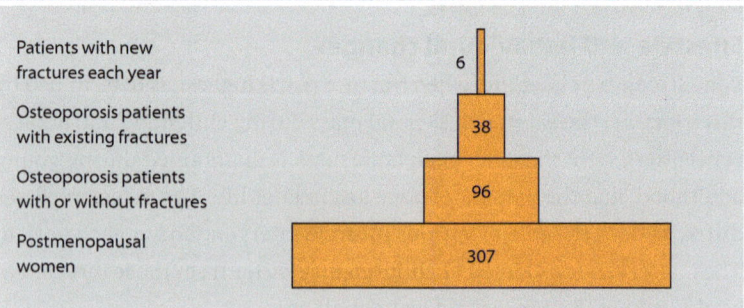

Osteoporosis and osteoporotic fractures: typical caseload for UK primary care practitioners

Patients with new fractures each year — 6

Osteoporosis patients with existing fractures — 38

Osteoporosis patients with or without fractures — 96

Postmenopausal women — 307

Figure 3.2 Osteoporosis and osteoporotic fractures: typical caseload for UK primary care practitioners. Assumes a total of 34,500 primary care practitioners with 1179 patients each. Data from Brown P. Improving practice – osteoporosis. Drugs in Context, October 2005.

Although firm evidence is lacking, other dietary and lifestyle recommendations may prove helpful in terms of reducing fracture risk. These include:

- avoid smoking,
- increase consumption of fruit and vegetables,
- reduce risk of falls (e.g. by correcting eye problems, avoiding slippery surfaces, installing adequate lighting),
- reduce impact of falls (e.g. by wearing hip protectors) and
- minimize glucocorticoid use.

The evidence supporting non-pharmacological approaches to the management of postmenopausal osteoporosis is discussed in Chapter 6.

Screening

The purpose of screening is to target interventions at those in need and avoid treating healthy individuals who have a low risk of disease, in this case fracture. There is no universally accepted policy for mass screening to identify people with osteoporosis. Because bone loss in women occurs at the menopause, the most obvious option would be to screen all perimenopausal women by means of bone densitometry and to use the level of bone mineral density (BMD) to estimate fracture risk. However this approach is not recommended, partly because of the poor long-term sensitivity and specificity of BMD measurement (the association between BMD and fracture is discussed in detail in Chapter 5) and also because, once patients at risk have been identified, long-term treatment with its associated costs would be required before any cost-saving on fractures would be achieved.

To achieve adequate sensitivity (i.e. a detection rate in the order of 90% or more) the specificity of BMD testing is low. If it is assumed that risk increases 1.5-fold for each standard deviation decrease in BMD, the sensitivity is only 18%. If a gradient of risk of 2.5 per standard deviation decrease is assumed, sensitivity is still only 34%. In this scenario, 1000 patients would need to be screened to detect 100 for treatment. If the treatment was assumed – optimistically – to be associated with 100% treatment compliance and 50% efficacy, this strategy would save 7% of hip fractures that would otherwise have occurred.

Another limitation of screening is poor long-term compliance with treatment. In the USA, for example, only around 10% of women continue taking hormone replacement therapy for more than 1 year [1]. Even with the introduction of weekly bisphosphonates, compliance after 12 months has risen from less than 40% to less than 60% [2]. Even when treatment is continued for extended periods, the ultimate effect depends not only on the effect induced, but also on the loss of effect when treatment is stopped. In terms of health economics therefore, screening all women at the menopause is not currently deemed to be cost-effective [3].

A more cost-effective approach to screening entails selecting higher risk individuals, and this might be achieved by screening women much older than 50 years. For example in the USA, the National Osteoporosis Foundation recommends measuring BMD in all white women aged 65 or older who are not receiving drugs approved for treating osteoporosis [4]. The guideline also suggests measuring BMD in younger postmenopausal women if they have another strong and well-established risk factor for osteoporosis. Similarly, the United States Preventive Services Task Force recommends routine screening starting at age 65 years in all women and at age 50 years in women with risk factors for osteoporotic fracture [5]. In contrast, a 2000 Consensus Development Conference sponsored by the US National Institutes of Health concluded that the value of universal osteoporosis screening was not yet established [6]. The conference panel recommended an individualized targeted approach, noting that bone density measurement is appropriate when it will aid the patient's decision to institute treatment.

Today, most countries do not endorse routine mass screening with bone densitometry for any subgroup of the population. However, there is interest in an approach that selects individuals at higher risk than is suggested on the basis of age or BMD alone. Combining BMD with other risk factors, such as clinical risk factors, biochemical markers or bone turnover, substantially increases the sensitivity of assessment without any loss of specificity (biochemical markers are discussed in Chapter 5). Under the auspices of the World Health Organization, a risk factor tool that has been developed that encompasses BMD assessment and clinical risk factors to determine 10-year risk of fracture (the FRAX tool [7]; see pp. 56–58). Risk assessment is discussed later in this chapter.

Targeted approaches

Case-finding strategies

Given the limitations associated with population-based strategies, the major thrust of osteoporosis prevention involves selective case-finding. This encompasses opportunistic identification of high-risk individuals and 'search and rescue' strategies for high-risk groups. Both approaches aim to identify people with fragility fractures or other strong risk factors for fracture and to refer them for further assessment, such as measurement of BMD. The indications for BMD measurement are discussed in Chapter 4.

Risk assessment

There is a growing view that the assessment of fracture risk should encompass all aspects of risk and that intervention should not be guided solely by BMD. Thus there is a distinction between diagnosis of osteoporosis and assessment of fracture risk, which in turn implies a distinction between diagnostic and intervention thresholds.

It is difficult to separate the risk factors for osteoporosis, falls and fracture, as the three are inextricably linked. Osteoporosis is itself a risk factor for fracture while, for example, a sedentary lifestyle contributes to osteoporosis risk and also to the risk of falling. While BMD is the strongest single risk factor for osteoporotic fracture, several other variables can predict fracture risk, some of which are independent of BMD.

Strong risk factors for osteoporosis and hence indications for BMD assessment include the following:
- previous fragility fracture (defined as a fracture),
- radiographic evidence of osteopaenia/vertebral deformity,
- loss of height, thoracic kyphosis (after radiographic confirmation of vertebral deformity),
- prolonged corticosteroid therapy (oral prednisolone for 3 months or more),

- premature menopause (<45 years),
- prolonged secondary amenorrhoea (>1 year),
- primary hypogonadism,
- maternal history of hip fracture,
- low body mass index (<19 kg/m^2) and
- other disorders associated with osteoporosis (e.g. anorexia nervosa, malabsorption syndromes, primary hyperparathyroidism, post transplantation, chronic renal failure, hyperthyroidism, Cushing syndrome and prolonged immobilization, and following transplantation).

Other risk factors for osteoporosis, falls and/or fracture include:
- female gender,
- reduced visual acuity,
- cigarette smoking,
- heavy alcohol intake (>3–4 units per day),
- inactivity,
- neuromuscular disorders,
- developmental disability,
- prolonged immobilization,
- Asian or Caucasian race and
- high bone turnover.

Risk assessment tools

A number of risk assessment tools have been developed to help clinicians identify women at increased risk of osteoporosis. Some of these have been prospectively validated in a broad spectrum of older women and are simple enough to use in the primary care setting; four such scores are described below.

As indicated above, the World Health Organization has now released a model that will allow prediction of 10-year fracture risk, similar to risk scoring for coronary heart disease [7].

Fracture Index

The Fracture Index was developed using data on 7782 women aged 65 years and older and has been validated in a separate group of 7575 French women [8]. The score includes seven items:

- age,
- BMD at the hip (optional),
- fracture after age 50 years,
- maternal hip fracture after age 50,
- weight ≤57 kg (125 lbs),
- smoking status, and
- the need to use the arms to stand up from a chair.

The Fracture Index can be used either with or without BMD testing to assess the 5-year risk of hip and other osteoporotic fractures. For hip fracture it has a sensitivity of 78.6 and specificity of 61.7%.

Fracture and Mortality Index

A new tool is the FRAMO (Fracture and Mortality) Index, which was validated in 1498 Swedish women aged 70 years and older [9]. It includes four items: age ≥80 years, weight <59.9 kg (132 lbs), previous fragility fracture (or vertebral compression seen on radiography), and the need to use the arms to rise from sitting. The FRAMO Index identifies high- and low-risk groups and predicts the 2-year risk of hip fracture and overall mortality (Figure 3.3). The FRAMO Index has 81% sensitivity and 64% specificity for predicting hip fracture, and 81% sensitivity and 67% specificity for predicting mortality.

Osteoporosis Risk Assessment Instrument

A third tool is the Osteoporosis Risk Assessment Instrument (ORAI), which was developed and validated using data on 1376 Canadian women aged 45 years or older [10]. The tool uses just three items: age, weight and current oestrogen use. It predicts low BMD with 93.3% sensitivity and 46.4% specificity, and predicts osteoporosis with 94.4% sensitivity. Using the ORAI substantially reduces the proportion of women who undergo bone densitometry.

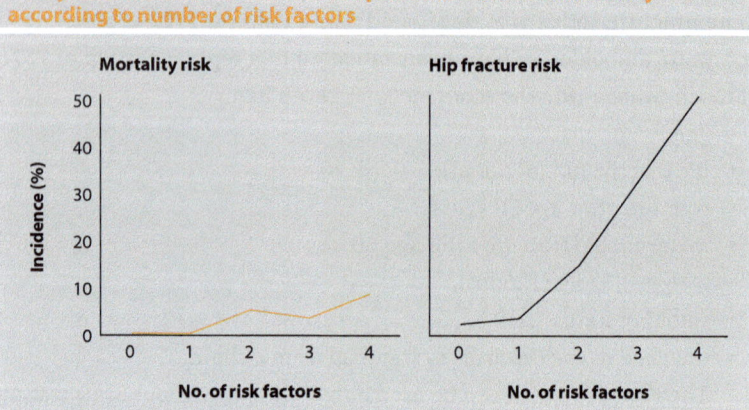

Figure 3.3 Two-year cumulative incidence of hip fracture and total mortality according to number of risk factors. Women were ≥80 years old, <60 kg, with ≤4 risk factors and previous fragility fracture, and using arms to rise. Proportions of women with 0, 1, 2, 3, and 4 risk factors were 30, 34, 22, 12, and 3%, respectively. Data from Albertsson et al [9].

Assessment by combining risk factors

In 1995 Cummings was among the first to identify the value of combining risk factors for prediction of hip fracture, Using information on 9516 white women aged 65 years and older, he identified 15 risk factors for hip fracture [11]:

- age > 80 years,
- fracture since the age of 50 years,
- maternal hip fracture,
- poor or very poor health,
- anticonvulsant treatment,
- long-acting benzodiazepine treatment,
- weight below that at the age of 25 years,
- height > 168 cm at the age of 25 years,
- consumption of more than two cups of coffee per day,
- on their feet for less than 4 hours per day,
- no walking for exercise,
- unable to rise from a chair without using their arms,
- previous hyperparathyroidism,

- lowest quartile depth perception,
- lowest quartile contrast sensitivity.

Women with five or more risk factors and calcaneal bone density in the lowest third for their age were 27 times more likely to suffer a hip fracture than those with two or fewer risk factors and (Figure 3.4).

References

1 Barrett-Connor E, Gore R, Browner WS, et al. Prevention of osteoporotic hip fracture: global versus high-risk strategies. Osteoporos Int 1998;8(suppl 1):S2–S7.

2 Cramer JA, Amonkar MM, Hebborn A, et al. Compliance and persistence with bisphosphonate dosing regimens among women with postmenopausal osteoporosis. Curr Med Res Opin 2005;21:1453–60.

3 World Health Organization (WHO). Prevention and management of osteoporosis. report of a WHO scientific group. WHO Technical Report Series 921. Geneva: WHO, 2003.

4 National Osteoporosis Foundation (NOF). Physician's guide to prevention and treatment of osteoporosis. Washington, DC: NOF; 1999.

5 US Preventive Services Task Force (USPSTF). Screening for osteoporosis in postmenopausal women: recommendations and rationale. Ann Intern Med 2002;137:526–8.

6 National Institutes of Health (NIH). Osteoporosis prevention, diagnosis, and therapy. NIH Consensus Statement Online 2000;17:1–36.

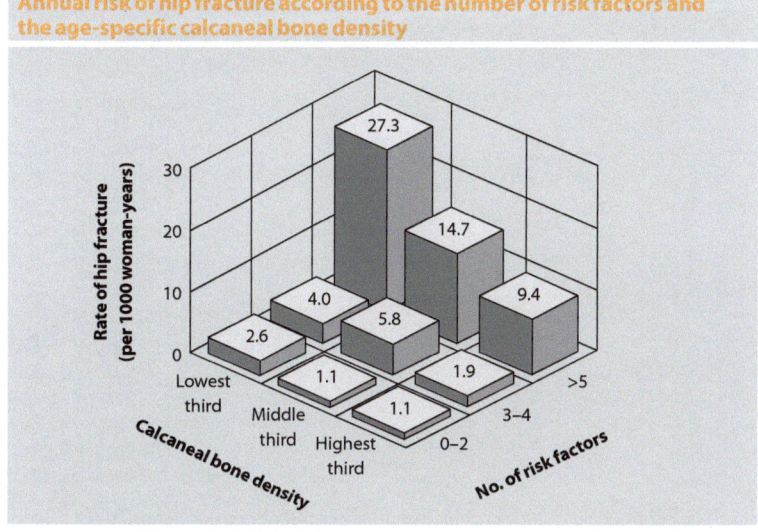

Annual risk of hip fracture according to the number of risk factors and the age-specific calcaneal bone density

Figure 3.4 Annual risk of hip fracture according to the number of risk factors and the age-specific calcaneal bone density. Reproduced with permission from Cummings SR, Nevitt MC, Browner WS, et al. Risk factors for hip fracture in white women. Study of Osteoporotic Fractures Research Group. N Engl J Med 1995;332:767–73. © 1995 Massachussetts Medical Society. All rights reserved.

7   Kanis JA, Johnell O, Oden A, Johansson H, McCloskey E. FRAX™ and the assessment of fracture probability in men and women from the UK. Osteoporos Int 2008;19:385–97.

8   Black DM, Steinbuch M, Palermo L, et al. An assessment tool for predicting fracture risk in postmenopausal women. Osteoporos Int 2001;12:519–28.

9   Albertsson DM, Mellström D, Petersson C, et al. Validation of a 4-item score predicting hip fracture and mortality risk among elderly women. Ann Fam Med 2007;5:48–56.

10 Cadarette SM, Jaglal SB, Kreiger N, et al. Development and validation of the Osteoporosis Risk Assessment Instrument to facilitate selection of women for bone densitometry. CMAJ 2000;162:1289–94.

11 Cummings SR, Nevitt MC, Browner WS, et al. Risk factors for hip fracture in white women. Study of Osteoporotic Fractures Research Group. N Engl J Med 1995;332:767–73.

Chapter 4

Investigation and diagnosis

Definition and diagnostic criteria

Osteoporosis literally means 'porous bone'. The definition of osteoporosis accepted at an international development conference in 2001 is that it is a skeletal disorder characterized by compromised bone strength predisposing a person to an increased risk of fracture. Bone strength reflects the integration of bone density and bone quality [1]. This description provides the framework for an operational definition based on measurement of bone mineral density (BMD) as there is no agreed methodology for assessing bone quality in vivo.

In 1994, a Study Group of the World Health Organization defined osteoporosis in women as a BMD 2.5 standard deviations (SD) or more below the average for the young healthy female population [2]. The Group defined three other categories: normal, low bone mass (osteopaenia), and severe (established) osteoporosis (Figure 4.1). In order to standardize values from different densitometers, densitometry results are reported

Osteoporosis: World Health Organization diagnostic categories		
Diagnosis	**Bone mineral density**	**T-score**
Normal	<1 SD below the young adult reference mean	≥−1
Osteopaenia	1–2.5 SD below the young adult mean	−1 to −2.5
Osteoporosis	>2.5 SD below the young adult mean	≤2.5
Severe (established) osteoporosis	>2.5 SD below young adult mean plus one or more fragility fractures	≤2.5

Figure 4.1 Osteoporosis: World Health Organization diagnostic categories. Bone mineral density and T-scores differ by site/method of measurement. SD, standard deviation. Data from World Health Organization [2].

as T scores, a T score being the number of SD above or below the value for young healthy adults of the same sex.

Using the WHO criteria, around 15% of the young healthy female population have low bone mass, or osteopaenia, and approximately 0.6% have osteoporosis. Since BMD in the population follows a normal distribution (Figure 4.2), the proportion of women with osteoporosis increases markedly with age, rising to 30–40% after the menopause.

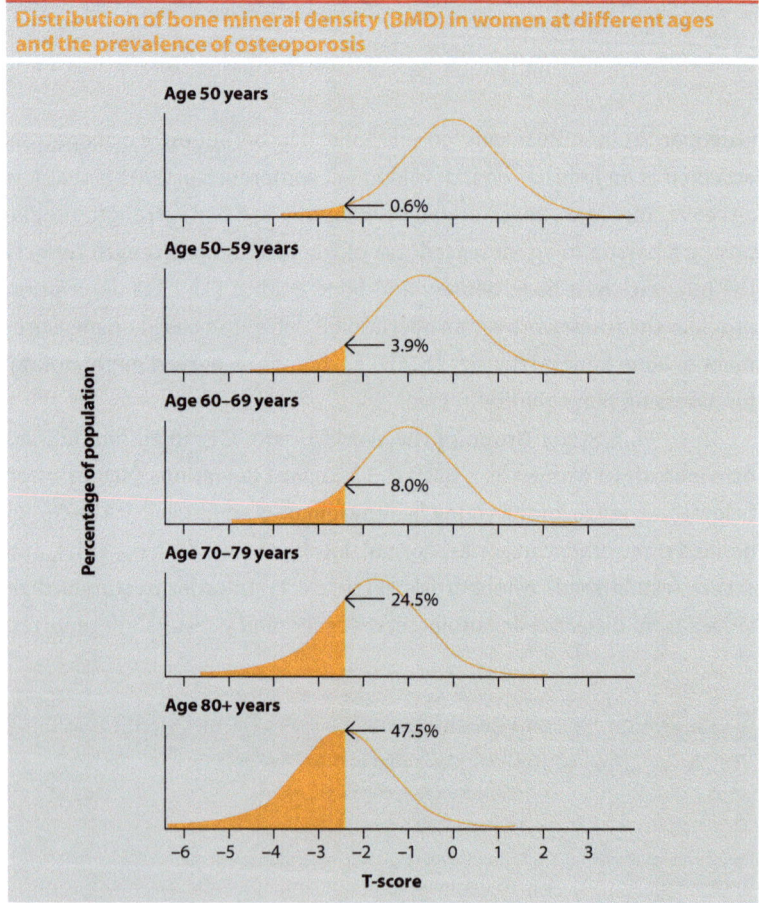

Distribution of bone mineral density (BMD) in women at different ages and the prevalence of osteoporosis

Figure 4.2 Distribution of bone mineral density (BMD) in women at different ages and the prevalence of osteoporosis at the hip. Reproduced from Kanis JA et al. The diagnosis of osteoporosis. J Bone Mineral Res 1994; 9:1137–41. With permission of the American Society for Bone and Mineral Research.

Assessment of osteoporosis

All postmenopausal women should be assessed for risk factors associated with osteoporosis. The assessment requires a history, physical examination, and diagnostic tests.

History and physical examination

History-taking and physical examination are important for detecting risk factors for osteoporosis and fracture (particularly modifiable risk factors); for identifying potential signs of established osteoporosis; and for ruling out secondary causes of osteoporosis (Figures 4.3 and 4.4). History and physical examination alone are not sufficient to diagnose osteoporosis, however.

Common secondary causes of bone loss
Medications
Glucocorticoids (e.g. prednisone) for >6 months
Excessive thyroxine doses
Long-term use of certain anticonvulsants (e.g. phenytoin)
Anticoagulants (e.g. heparin, warfarin)
Cytotoxic agents
Gonadotropin-releasing hormone agonists or analogues
Intramuscular medroxyprogesterone contraceptive
Immunosuppressives (e.g. cyclosporin)
Aromatase inhibitors for breast cancer
Androgen deprivation therapy for prostate cancer
Proton-pump inhibitors
Thiazolidinediones
Genetic disorders
Haemophilia
Thalassaemia
Hypophosphatasia
Haemachromatosis
Homocystinuria
Disorders of calcium balance
Hypercalciura
Vitamin D deficiency

Figure 4.3 Common secondary causes of bone loss (continues overleaf).

Common secondary causes of bone loss (continued)

Endocrinopathies

Cortisol excess

Cushing syndrome

Gonadal insufficiency (primary and secondary)

Hyperthyroidism

Type 1 diabetes mellitus

Primary hyperarathyroidism

Gastrointestinal diseases

Chronic liver disease (e.g. primary biliary cirrhosis)

Malabsorption syndromes (e.g. coeliac disease, Crohn's disease)

Total gastrectomy

Billroth 1 gastroenterostomy

Other disorders and conditions

Multiple myeloma

Lymphoma and leukaemia

Systemic mastocytosis

Nutritional disorders (e.g. anorexia nervosa)

Rheumatoid arthritis

Chronic renal disease

Figure 4.3 Common secondary causes of bone loss (continued). Adapted with permission from North American Menopause Society (NAMS). Management of postmenopausal osteoporosis: position statement of the North American Menopause Society. Menopause 2002;9:84–101.

Routine laboratory tests for evaluation of osteoporosis

Test	Diagnostic result	Possible secondary cause
Complete blood cell count	Anaemia	Multiple myeloma
Serum calcium	Elevated	Hyperparathyroidism
	Low	Vitamin D deficiency, malabsorption
Serum alkaline phosphatase	Elevated	Vitamin D deficiency, malabsorption, hyperparathyroidism
Serum albumin	Used to interpret serum calcium	
Urinary calcium excretion	Elevated	Renal calcium leak, multiple myeloma, metastatic bone cancer, hyperparathyroidism, hyperthyroidism
	Low	Malabsorption, vitamin D deficiency
Thyroid-stimulating hormone	Low	Hyperthyroidism
Endomyseal antibodies	Positive	Coeliac disease

Figure 4.4 Routine laboratory tests for evaluation of osteoporosis. Reproduced with permission from North American Menopause Society (NAMS). Management of postmenopausal osteoporosis: position statement of the North American Menopause Society. Menopause 2002;9:84–101.

Osteoporosis is often described as a 'silent' disease because around half of patients are asymptomatic. Nevertheless the condition may manifest in physical signs. For example, loss of height can indicate the presence of one or more vertebral compression fractures (Figure 4.5). Height should be measured using an accurate and precise method, such as by use of a stadiometer.

Acute or chronic back pain is another symptom of vertebral fracture. The mid-back vertebrae, T12 and L1, are the most common fractures sites, followed by T6 to T9 [3]. Multiple compression fractures ultimately lead to the most obvious sign of osteoporosis, kyphosis (abnormal curvature of the thoracic spine). Because back pain, height loss and kyphosis can occur without osteoporosis, the presence of vertebral fractures should be confirmed by radiography (Figure 4.6).

Clinical investigations

A variety of methods can be used to investigate fracture risk in postmenopausal women. The most common diagnostic approaches are listed in Figure 4.7 and described in more detail below.

Vertebral fracture between two osteoporotic vertebrae

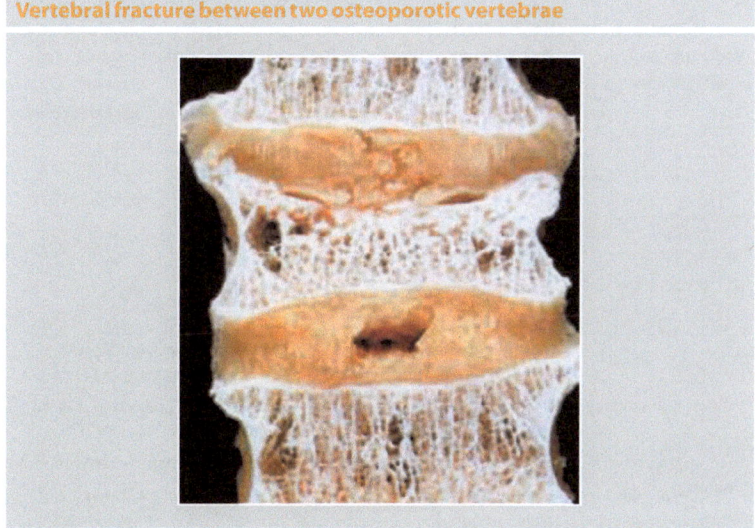

Figure 4.5 Vertebral fracture between two osteoporotic vertebrae. Reproduced with permission from Rizzoli R, Atlas of Postmenopausal Osteoporosis, 2nd edition, London: Current Medicine Group Limited, 2005.

Vertebral fractures

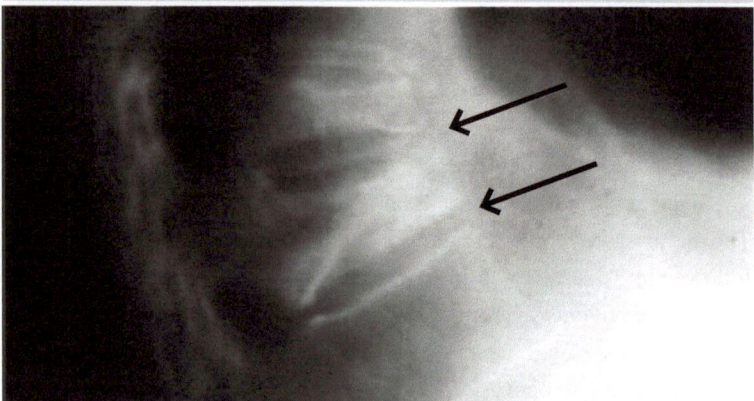

Figure 4.6 Vertebral fracture (arrows). By courtesy of Professor Stuart Ralston, University of Edinburgh.

Diagnosis of postmenopausal osteoporosis: summary of techniques and their advantages and drawbacks

Bone densitometry	'Gold standard' in diagnosis of osteoporosis
	Primarily a quantitative measurement technique for assessing BMD (rather than imaging technique)
	Measuring changes in BMD can be used to assess efficacy of therapeutic agents
Radiography	Plain radiographs only enable visualization of advanced osteoporosis (BMD reduction at least 30–50%)
	Normal appearance on a plain radiograph does not exclude osteoporosis
	Evaluation of bone density from plain radiographs is subject to significant observer variation
	Enables confirmation of osteoporotic fracture
	Useful technique for exclusion of diseases which may be associated with back or limb pain, e.g. osteoarthritis or Paget's disease
Bone scan	May reveal a recent vertebral fracture that is not revealed by plain radiography
	May help to exclude other causes of bone pain in individuals with osteoporosis, e.g. metastatic bone disease or Paget's disease
Isotope bone biopsy	Useful in unusual cases of osteoporosis and when coexisting disease suspected, e.g. secondary tumour or osteomalacia
Magnetic resonance imaging	May indicate sites of recent fracture by revealing marrow oedema
	Enables diagnosis of insufficiency fractures that do not show up on plain radiographs, e.g. fractures of sacrum

Figure 4.7 Diagnosis of postmenopausal osteoporosis: summary of techniques and their advantages and drawbacks.

Densitometry

The most widely used technique to measure BMD is bone densitometry, which assesses the amount of mineral present per unit area as a guide to bone strength. BMD measurements may be performed for diagnostic purposes, to diagnose osteoporosis or osteopaenia; for monitoring purposes, to assess changes in BMD over time and in response to treatment; and for risk assessment, to predict the risk of fracture.

Although bone density can be measured in absolute terms (g/cm^2), the results are more meaningful if given in relative terms. As described at the start of this chapter, the T-score is the patient's BMD relative to the average BMD in a young healthy adult of the same sex. The Z-score is the patient's BMD relative to the average BMD in a healthy person of the same age, sex, and ethnic origin. T- and Z-scores are based on the use of a normative range, which should be a standard based on the National Health and Nutrition Examination Survey NHANES III for hip measurements and well developed manufacturer's normative ranges for the lumbar spine [4].

Several densitometry technologies are used, including (Figure 4.8):

- dual-energy X-ray absorptiometry (DXA),
- peripheral or single-X-ray densitometry (pDXA/SXA),
- quantitative computed tomography (QCT), and
- quantitative ultrasound (QUS).

DXA can be used to measure BMD in the axial (central) skeleton and at appendicular (peripheral) sites, such as the wrist or heel, and to measure the bone mineral content of the entire skeleton. It is the 'gold standard' investigation for diagnosing osteoporosis (see later): a T-score ≤ 2.5 based on DXA of the axial (central) skeleton, usually measured at the hip or spine, is the WHO diagnostic criteria for osteoporosis.

The hip – either the femoral neck or total hip region of interest (ROI) – is the preferred site for DXA for diagnostic purposes, particularly in elderly individuals, because of its high predictive value for fracture risk (Figure 4.9): risk increases approximately 2-fold for each SD increase in BMD. Hip BMD is unaffected by degenerative changes. and has many other advantages, including high precision and accuracy, high resolution, a quick scan time, and a very low radiation dose.

The drawbacks of DXA are that it combines trabecular and cortical measurements; it provides a two-dimensional areal value rather than a volumetric density and thus gives no indication of bone quality; and spine DXA measurements may be influenced by degenerative changes and other artefacts.

Peripheral DXA and single-energy X-ray absorptiometry can also be helpful in identifying patients at high risk of fracture. These approaches measure bone density in the forearm or heel and are predictive of site-specific fracture and offer some predictive information about hip and spine fractures.

Densitometry techniques

Dual-energy radiograph absorptiometry (DXA)	Two-dimensional measurements of bone density of cortical and trabecular bone (can not differentiate between the two types of bone)
	Used to measure bone mineral content:
	• of whole skeleton
	• at specific sites at high risk of fracture
	Most versatile densitometry technique
	Most effective way of estimating risk of postmenopausal fracture in Caucasian women
Quantitative computed tomography (QCT)	Three-dimensional measurements of bone density in which cortical and trabecular bone can be separated
	Useful for measurement of vertebral bone density, but in clinical practice has not been adapted for proximal femur measurement
	Less precise and more expensive than DXA
	Higher radiation exposure than DXA
	Mainly a research tool; but is best non-invasive tool for measuring trabecular volumetric density
Quantitative ultrasound (QUS)	Measures speed and attenuation of sound as it passes through bone:
	• Speed is related to the density and quality of the bone
	• Attenuation is related to bone density and architecture
	Most QUS devices measure bone mass in the heel
	Used to predict fracture risk
	Not used to diagnose osteoporosis or assess efficacy of antiresorptive agents because QUS results correlate poorly with BMD measurements and there are no population standards
Radiographic absorptiometry (RA)	A region of the distal appendicular skeleton and an aluminium wedge known density are simultaneously exposed to a radiographic beam and the densities compared
Radiogrammetry (radiographic morphometry)	Internal and external dimensions of the bones are measured with fine callipers from plain radiographs or by automated means using digitized images, usually of the hand

Figure 4.8 Densitometry techniques. BMD, bone mineral density. Data from Bonnick [5].

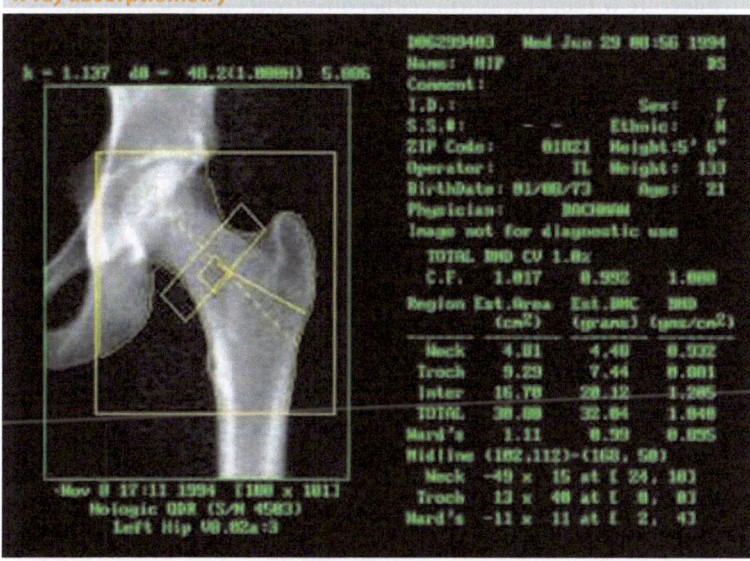

Figure 4.9 Proximal femur bone mineral density measurement by dual-energy X-ray absorptiometry. Reproduced with permission from Rizzoli R, Atlas of Postmenopausal Osteoporosis, 2nd edition, London: Current Medicine Group Limited, 2005.

In order to visualize the bone microarchitecture, researchers and clinicians are increasingly turning to newer techniques. QCT is unique because it assesses three-dimensional bone density and permits isolated measurement of trabecular and cortical bone. This makes it particularly useful for assessing effects of treatment on cortical porosity for example, hence its application as a research tool. The value of QCT measurements for prediction of fractures has not been well studied, however. Compared with DXA, QCT is more sensitive but less precise and much more expensive. It is also associated with much higher radiation exposure.

Bone mass can also be measured using QUS, which differs from routine clinical ultrasound imaging techniques. The transmission of sound through bone reflects its density and structure and can be assessed quantitatively by the speed of sound (SOS), the pattern of absorption of different wavelengths of sound (called broadband ultrasound attenuation, BUA), or calculations derived from these parameters (Figure 4.10).

QUS thus allows an assessment of bone which encompasses density and architecture without measuring either directly. It offers insights into skeletal status and fragility that can not be measured using absorptiometric techniques alone, although there remains uncertainty as to exactly which parameters are being measured.

QUS is usually performed at the heel as a way of assessing hip and overall fracture risk. Most studies suggest that measurement of SOS or BUA are associated with a 1.5- to 2-fold increase in fracture risk for each SD decrease in SOS, BUA or their integrals. These gradients of risk are very similar to those provided by assessment of peripheral BMD by absorptiometric techniques to predict any osteoporotic fracture. Indeed the combination of calcaneal BUA and femoral neck BMD predicts hip fracture risk better than either measurement alone [6].

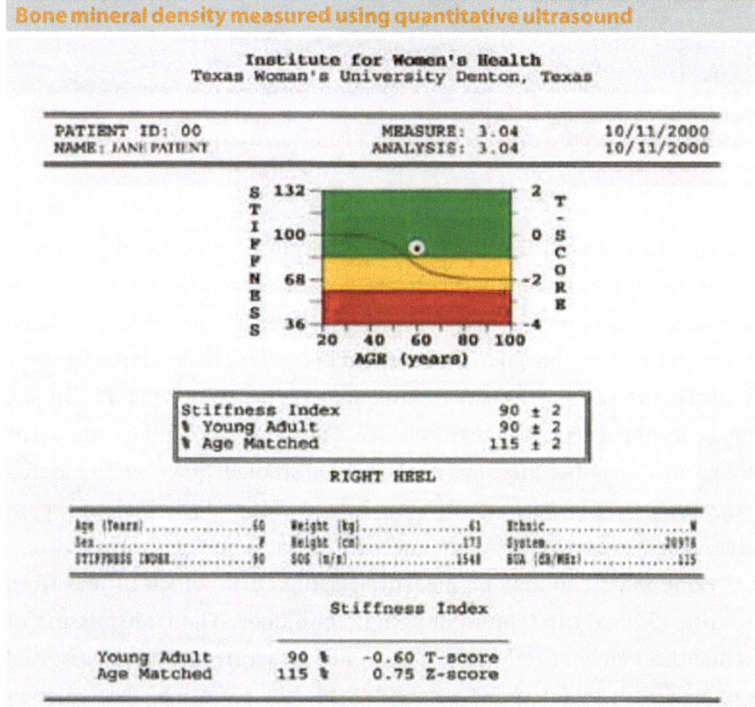

Figure 4.10 Bone mineral density measured using quantitative ultrasound. Reproduced with permission from Rizzoli R, Atlas of Postmenopausal Osteoporosis, 2nd edition, London: Current Medicine Group Limited, 2005.

QUS is relatively inexpensive and entails no radiation exposure. It may be useful for fracture risk assessment; however, it cannot be used for the diagnosis of osteoporosis or assessing the response to therapy.

Radiography

In Europe, radiography is used to assess and confirm osteoporotic fractures (Figure 4.11), to suggest the presence of osteopaenia (Figure 4.12), and to monitor the progression of osteoporotic fractures over time (Figure 4.13). Radiography is also used in the investigation of back or limb pain to exclude diseases such as osteoarthritis or Paget's disease.

In areas of the world where DXA is not available, radiography is widely used to diagnose osteoporosis. However a normal appearance on a plain radiograph does not exclude osteoporosis and the evaluation of bone density is subject to significant observer variation. A decrease in radiographic bone density is more appropriately termed osteopaenia.

Radiograph showing Colles' fracture of the wrist

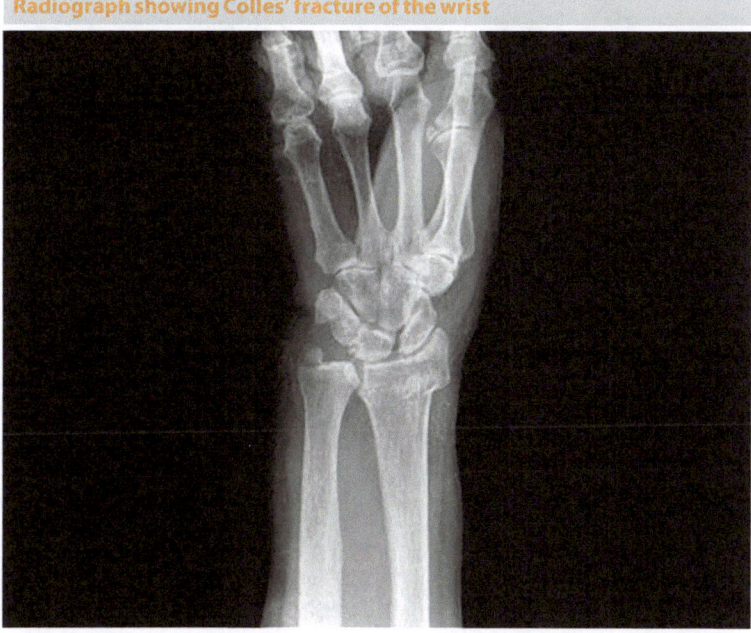

Figure 4.11 Radiograph showing Colles' fracture of the wrist and fracture of the tip of the ulna. Reproduced with permission from Rizzoli R, Atlas of Postmenopausal Osteoporosis, 2nd edition, London: Current Medicine Group Limited, 2005.

The Genant SQ method is a semiquantitative method for assessing vertebral fractures in people with osteoporosis and has been extensively used in clinical trials and epidemiological research [7]. It uses visual inspection of vertebral radiographs to assign grades to each vertebra based on the approximate degree of height reduction and morphological changes (Figure 4.14). The result is a 'spinal deformity index'.

In specific circumstances, techniques such as bone scintigraphy, magnetic resonance imaging, or bone biopsy are used to investigate osteoporosis.

Radiography of the lumbar spine showing osteopaenia

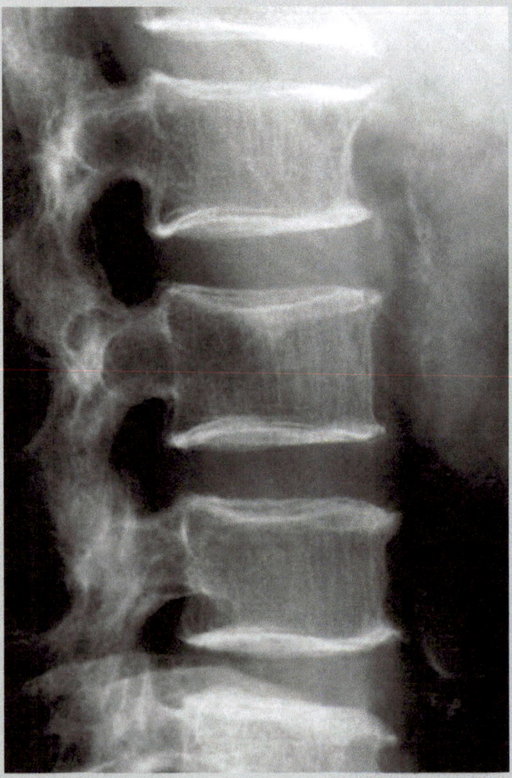

Figure 4.12 Radiography of the lumbar spine showing osteopaenia. Reproduced with permission from Rizzoli R, Atlas of Postmenopausal Osteoporosis, 2nd edition, London: Current Medicine Group Limited, 2005.

The gold standard for diagnosis

The internationally accepted gold standard for diagnosis of osteoporosis is measurement of BMD using axial DXA at the femoral neck or total hip ROI. The result should be interpreted according to the WHO criteria in Figure 4.1 and using a T-score calculated from an appropriate reference range.

Importantly, DXA is indicated only when the results would change the subsequent management of the patient. In the United Kingdom, for example, the National Insitute of Health and Clinical Excellence (NICE) guidance states that women aged 75 years and over who have already suffered an osteoporotic fragility fracture do not require a DXA scan before starting bone-sparing therapy [8].

The indications for measurement of BMD as defined by the UK Royal College of Physicians and the United States National Osteoporosis Foundation, respectively, are shown in Figure 4.15 [9,10].

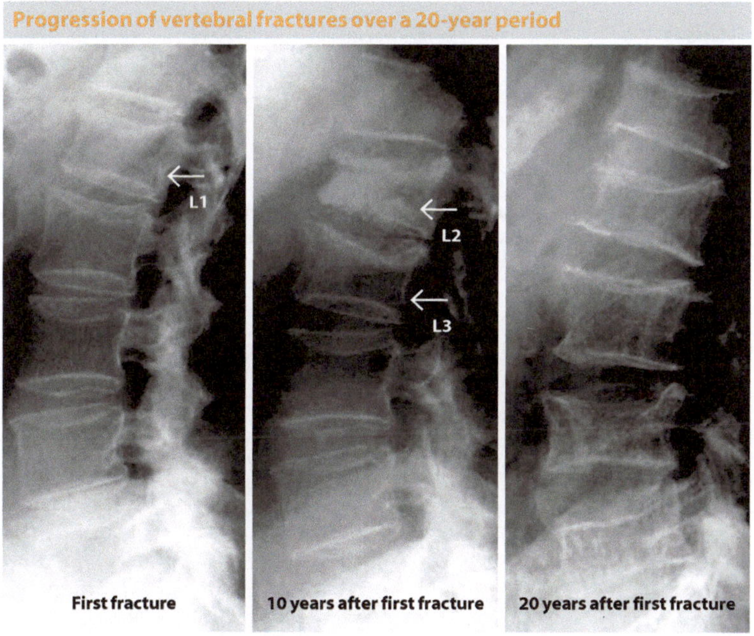

Progression of vertebral fractures over a 20-year period

First fracture | 10 years after first fracture | 20 years after first fracture

Figure 4.13 Progression of vertebral fractures over a 20-year period. Reproduced with permission from Rizzoli R, Atlas of Postmenopausal Osteoporosis, 2nd edition, London: Current Medicine Group Limited, 2005.

Genant semiquantitative method for grading vertebral fractures

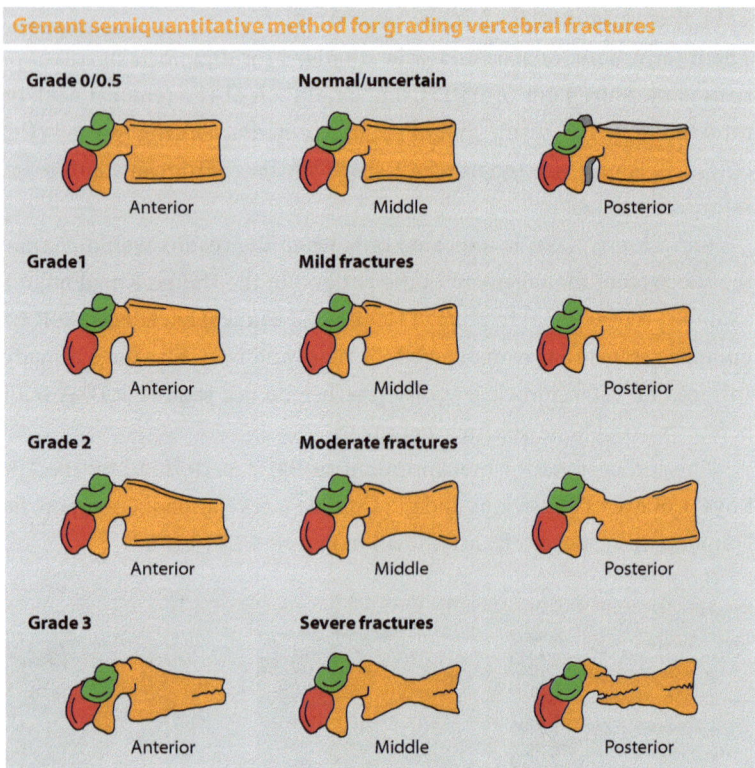

Figure 4.14 Genant semiquantitative method for grading vertebral fractures. Reproduced with permission from Genant HK, Jergas M. Assessment of prevalent and incident vertebral fractures in osteoporosis research. Osteoporos Int 2003; 14(Suppl 3):S43–S55.

Indications for measurement of bone mineral density

US (National Osteoporosis Foundation)	UK (Royal College of Physicians)
• All women aged 65 and older regardless of risk factors • Younger postmenopausal women ≥ 1 more risk factors • Postmenopausal women who present with fractures	• Radiographic osteopaenia • Vertebral deformity • Previous fragility fracture • Prolonged corticosteroids • Premature menopause • Prolonged amenorrhoea • Primary hypogonadism • Other diseases associated with osteoporosis • Maternal history of hip fracture • Low body mass index

Figure 4.15 Indications for measurement of bone mineral density. Data from Royal College of Physicians [9] and National Osteoporosis [10].

References

1   NIH Consensus Development Panel on Osteoporosis Prevention, Diagnosis, and Therapy. Consensus panel on osteoporosis prevention. 2001. JAMA 2001; 285:785–95.

2   World Health Organization (WHO). Assessment of fracture risk and its application to screening for postmenopausal osteoporosis. WHO Technical Report Series 843. Geneva: WHO, 1994.

3   Wasnich RD. Vertebral fracture epidemiology. Bone 1996;18:179–83S.

4   Blake GM, Fogelman I. Role of dual-energy X-ray absorptiometry in the diagnosis and treatment of osteoporosis. J Clin Densitom 2007;10:102-10

5   Bonnick SL. Pocket Reference to Bone Densitometry. New York: Science Press Inc, 2001.

6   Cummings SR, Bates D, Black DM. Clinical use of bone densitometry: scientific review. JAMA 2002;288:1889–97.

7   Genant HK, Jergas M. Assessment of prevalent and incident vertebral fractures in osteoporosis research. Osteoporos Int 2003;14 (suppl 3):S43–55.

8   National Institute for Health and Clinical Excellence (NICE). Bisphosphonates (alendronate, etidronate, risedronate), selective oestrogen receptor modulators (raloxifene) and parathyroid hormone (teriparatide) for the secondary prevention of osteoporotic fragility fractures in postmenopausal women. Technology Appraisal 87. London: NICE; January 2005.

9   Royal College of Physicians. Osteoporosis: clinical guidelines for prevention and treatment. London: Royal College of Physicians; 1999.

10 National Osteoporosis Foundation (NOF). Physician's guide to prevention and treatment of osteoporosis. Washington, DC: NOF; 1999.

Chapter 5

Fracture risk assessment

BMD and fracture risk

Osteoporotic fractures result from decreased bone mineral mass, changes to bone microarchitecture or geometry, and/or low-energy trauma as a result of loss of balance, inappropriate protective responses, or muscle weakness (Figure 5.1). Bone mineral density (BMD) is a strong predictor of fracture risk because bone mass accounts for 75–85% of the variation in bone strength [1]. Additional factors that contribute to fracture risk include other bone abnormalities and non-skeletal factors such as the liability to fall and the force of the impact.

The association between BMD and fracture risk has been established in prospective observational studies. A meta-analysis of 11 such studies, with around 90,000 person-years of observation and over 2000 fractures, found that the risk of fracture increases progressively with decreasing BMD (Marshall et al. 1996). Importantly, there was no BMD threshold below which fracture risk abruptly increased. Instead BMD is a continuous risk factor, whereby the lower the BMD the higher the risk of fracture.

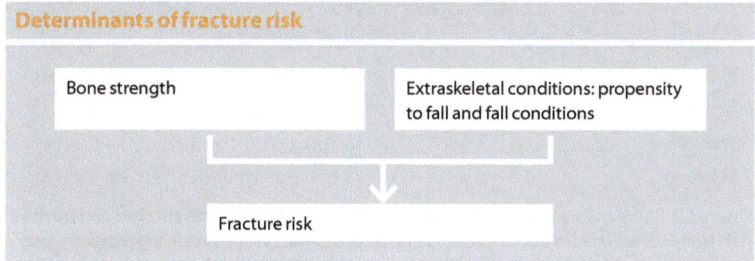

Figure 5.1 Determinants of fracture risk. Reproduced with permission from Rizzoli R. Atlas of Postmenopausal Osteoporosis, 2nd edition. London: Current Medicine Group Limited, 2005.

In the meta-analysis by Marshall et al., when BMD was measured at any site, the relative risk of fracture rose 1.5-fold for each 1 standard deviation (SD) decrease in BMD below the age-adjusted mean. The analysis also found that the predictive accuracy of BMD measurements was site dependent; the relative risks of fracture associated with a 1 SD decrease in BMD at the spine and hip were 2.3 and 2.6, respectively [2]. To put these values in context, the ability of BMD to predict fracture is equivalent to blood pressure in predicting stroke, and substantially better than blood cholesterol in predicting coronary heart disease [3].

The predictive ability of BMD was confirmed in a recent review of meta-analyses, systematic reviews and other prospective data sets [4]. This review confirmed that BMD predicts fracture risk and that hip BMD is the best predictor of hip fracture (Figure 5.2). However it also showed that hip and spine BMD are similarly accurate in predicting vertebral fractures, and that all anatomical sites and types of measurements have similar accuracy in predicting the general risk of all fractures.

BMD can also be used in combination with age to estimate the absolute fracture risk in postmenopausal white women (Figure 5.3). Currently there are insufficient data to translate BMD results into absolute fracture risks for non-white women.

Swedish population data have been used to predict the 10-year risk of osteoporotic fractures of the hip, spine and forearm at different ages and levels of BMD [5]. With the exception of forearm fractures in men, fracture risk increased with decreasing BMD and increasing age.

Relationship between bone mineral density (BMD) at different sites and fracture risk

BMD measurement site	Type of fracture (95% CI)			
	Hip	Vertebral	Forearm	All
Hip	2.4 (2.2–2.6)	1.9 (1.8–2.1)	1.4 (1.4–1.6)	1.6 (1.4–1.8)
Lumbar spine	1.5 (1.3–1.7)	1.9 (1.8–2.0)	1.5 (1.3–1.8)	1.5 (1.4–1.7)
Distal radius	1.5 (1.3–1.8)	1.7 (1.5–1.9)	1.7 (1.4–2.0)	1.4 (1.3–1.6)
Calcaneus	1.8 (1.5–2.1)	1.7 (1.5–1.9)	1.6 (1.4–1.8)	1.5 (1.4–1.6)

Figure 5.2 Relationship between bone mineral density (BMD) at different sites and fracture risk. Numbers are relative risk for fracture per standard deviation decrease in the measurement. CI, confidence interval. Reproduced with permission from Cummings SR, Bates D, Black DM. Clinical use of bone densitometry: scientific review. JAMA 2002;288:1889-97.

For example, over a 4 SD interval in BMD, the risk of hip fracture is increased 14-fold at the age of 50 years in women but 145-fold at the age of 80 years (Figure 5.4). For any given BMD the risk increases exponentially with increasing age. A similar phenomenon was observed in both sexes and for all fracture types.

Lifetime risk of hip fracture in white women in relation to femoral neck bone mineral density

Age (years)	Femoral neck bone mineral density T-score							
	−3.5	−3.0	−2.5	−2.0	−1.5	−1.0	−0.5	0
50	49	41	33	27	21	16	13	10
60	47	40	33	27	21	17	13	10
70	46	39	33	27	21	17	13	10
80	41	35	30	24	20	16	12	10

Figure 5.3 Lifetime risk of hip fracture in white women in relation to femoral neck bone mineral density. Reproduced with permission from Cummings SR, Bates D, Black DM. Clinical use of bone densitometry: scientific review. JAMA 2002;288:1889–97.

Relationship between women's bone mineral density at the hip and hip fracture risk according to age

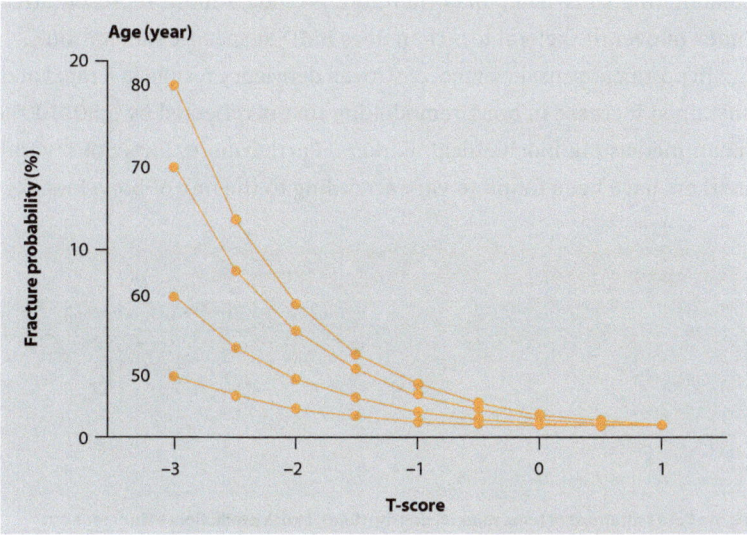

Figure 5.4 Relationship between women's bone mineral density at the hip and hip fracture risk according to age. For any given T-score the risk is higher with increasing age. Reproduced with permission from Kanis JA, Johnell O, Oden A, et al. Ten year probabilities of osteoporotic fractures according to BMD and diagnostic thresholds. Osteoporos Int 2001;12:989-95.

Limitations of BMD

BMD can predict fracture risk but can not identify individuals who will suffer a fracture. In other words, there is wide overlap between the BMD values of patients who develop a fracture and those who do not. In their meta-analysis, Marshall et al. calculated the sensitivity, specificity, positive predictive value and population-attributable risk for a cut-off point in BMD of 1 SD below the age-adjusted mean [2]. The values associated with three different lifetime incidences of hip fracture are shown in Figure 5.5. The sensitivity and population-attributable risk decreased with increasing lifetime incidence of fractures. Thus, the majority of all fractures would occur in women with a negative test. The low sensitivity of BMD is one of the reasons why population-based screening is not recommended in women at the time of the menopause [6].

Biochemical markers of bone turnover

Biochemical markers reflect systemic rates of bone resorption and bone formation and are thought to reflect changes in the number of bone remodelling sites. They may therefore provide a more representative index of overall skeletal loss than does BMD at specific skeletal sites.

In postmenopausal women, oestrogen deficiency results in a rapid and sustained increase in bone remodelling that is reflected by a 50–100% mean increase in biochemical markers. Furthermore, levels of several markers have been found to vary according to the rate of bone loss [7].

Limitations of bone mineral density (BMD) in risk prediction: values for a cut-off point in BMD of 1 SD below age-adjusted mean

	Lifetime incidence of hip fracture (%)		
	3	15	30
Sensitivity (%)	47	37	34
Specificity (%)	83	88	89
Positive predictive value (%)	9	36	58
Population-attributable risk (%)	36	26	21

Figure 5.5 Limitations of bone mineral density (BMD) in risk prediction: values for a cut-off point in BMD of 1 SD below age-adjusted mean. Relative risk of hip fracture is assumed to be 2.6 per 1 SD decrease in bone density. Reproduced with permission from Marshall D, Johnell O, Wedel H. Meta-analysis of how well measures of bone mineral density predict occurrence of osteoporotic fractures. BMJ 1996;312:1254–9.

This has led to interest in using biochemical markers to help to determine fracture risk and to assess the response to therapy.

The markers listed in Figure 5.6 are more sensitive than conventional markers of bone turnover, such as total alkaline phosphate. They can be divided into two categories: those for measuring bone formation and those for measuring bone resorption. Some may reflect both mechanisms.

It is important to note that these markers are not disease specific and will measure alterations in skeletal metabolism regardless of the underlying cause. The markers of bone formation detect direct or indirect products of active osteoblasts, which are expressed at different phases of development, and reflect osteoblast function and bone formation. These markers are measured in the serum, or plasma. The markers for bone resorption are generally degradation products of collagen, but markers for non-collagenous proteins are also being investigated [7].

Biochemical markers and fracture risk

The relationship between biochemical markers of bone turnover and fracture risk have been investigated in several prospective studies. The evidence concerning markers of bone formation and fracture risk is conflicting, although markers of bone resorption have been generally linked with fracture risk. One study found that women classified as 'fast bone losers' within 3 years of menopause were twice as likely to sustain spine or peripheral fractures during 15 years of follow-up than were 'normal' or 'slow" losers [8]. In this study, a low BMD conferred the same magnitude of fracture risk as did a high rate of bone loss at the radius. Furthermore, women with both risk factors had a higher likelihood of fracture than those with only one of the two factors.

Similar results have been obtained in four major prospective studies, indicating that increased levels of bone resorption markers are associated with an increased risk of hip, vertebral, non-hip and non-vertebral fracture over follow-up periods of 1.8–5 years. The predictive value is consistently in the order of a 2-fold increase in fracture risk for levels above the upper limit of the premenopausal range. Unlike BMD, increased bone resorption is associated with an increased risk of fracture only for values above a threshold [7].

Markers for assessing bone formation and resorption

Formation markers	Comments about assay
Osteocalcin	
Osteocalcin (or bone-Gla-protein [BGP])	
Undercarboxylated osteocalcin	
Total osteocalcin	Intact + N-mid fragment
Intact osteocalcin	
N-mid fragment of osteocalcin	
Alkaline phosphatase	
Total alkaline phosphatase	Bone + liver + other sources
Bone specific alkaline phosphatase	
Type 1 collagen propeptides*	
Procollagen type 1 N propeptide	
Monomer of procollagen type 1	
N propeptide	
Intact procollagen type 1 N propeptide	Monomer + trimer
Total procollagen type 1 N propeptide	
Procollagen type 1 C propeptide	
Resorption markers	
Hydroxyproline Hydroxylysine }	Total (ie, free + peptide-bound) urinary excretion unless otherwise specified
Galactosyl hydroxylysine Glucosyl galactosyl hydroxylysine }	Urinary excretion of free moieties unless otherwise specified
Pyridinoline Deoxypyridinoline }	Can be qualified by total, free moieties or peptide-bound and in serum and urine
Type 1 collagen telopeptides	
N-terminal cross-linking telopeptide of type 1 collagen	
C-terminal cross-linking telopeptide of type 1 collagen	Beta isomerized unless otherwise specified
C-terminal cross-linking telopeptide of type 1 collagen generated by matrix metalloproteinases	
Bone sialoprotein	
Acid phosphatase	
Tartrate-resistant acid phosphatase	Includes two isoforms: type 5a (platelets and other sources) and type 5b (osteoclasts)

*Also called extension peptides of type 1 collagen. Refers to trimer

Figure 5.6 Markers for assessing bone formation and resorption. Reproduced with permission from Delmas PD, Eastell R, Garnero P, et al. The use of biochemical markers of bone turnover in osteoporosis. Osteoporosis Int 2000; 11(suppl 6):S2–S17.

Combining BMD and biochemical markers

Since bone resorption markers may predict fracture risk independently of BMD, the two tests may be combined to improve the identification of women at high risk of fracture. Data from a large prospective study, the Epidemiology of Osteoporosis Study (EPIDOS), showed that combining a bone resorption marker with hip BMD could detect women at very high risk of fracture. Women with low hip BMD and high bone resorption had a 4- to 5-fold increased risk compared with the general population [9]. The utility of this approach has also been confirmed for other fracture sites (Figure 5.7) [10]. By using such a combination, the specificity of hip fracture prediction is increased without a loss of sensitivity [7].

While these data are encouraging, the routine use of biochemical markers to help predict future fracture risk is not featured in most management guidelines.

Combination of BMD and bone turnover markers to predict fracture risk in postmenopausal women

	Odds ratio* (95% CI)	Likelihood ratio	Probability of fracture over 5 years (%)
All women	–	–	12.6
Low femoral neck BMD (T-score ≤–2.5)	2.8 (1.4–5.6)	1.70	39
High bone resorption			
• High S-CTX (T-score ≥2)	2.1 (1.2–3.8)	1.70	25
• High U-free DPD (T-score ≥2)	1.8 (1.0–3.4)	1.68	24
Low BMD + high CTX	3.8 (1.9–7.3)	3.70	54
Low BMD + high free DPD	2.1 (0.7–6.2)	3.04	45

*Adjusted for age, prevalent fractures and physical activity

Figure 5.7 Combination of BMD and bone turnover markers to predict fracture risk in postmenopausal women. Four hundred and thirty-five healthy untreated postmenopausal women (mean age 64 years, range 50–89 years) were followed prospectively for an average of 5 years. During this follow-up period, 58 incident fractures (21 vertebral, 37 peripheral fractures) occurred in 55 women. The T-scores of BMD, S-CTX and free DPD were calculated from the mean and standard deviation of premenopausal women from the same cohort. BMD, Bone mineral density; S-CTX, serum C-terminal crosslinking telopeptide of type I collagen; U-free DPD, urinary free deoxypyridinoline. Reproduced with permission from Delmas PD, Eastell R, Garnero P, et al. The use of biochemical markers of bone turnover in osteoporosis. Osteoporosis Int 2000; 11(suppl 6):S2–S17.

Biochemical markers and treatment response

Monitoring the efficacy of osteoporosis treatment is a challenge. The goal of treatment is to reduce the occurrence of fragility fractures. Since the incidence of such fractures is so low, however, the absence of fractures following the initiation of treatment does not necessarily imply that treatment is effective. Although BMD has been widely used as a surrogate marker of treatment efficacy and in clinical trials, its usefulness in monitoring treatment in individual patients has not been well validated.

For patients being treated with antiresorptive agents (see Chapter 7), biochemical markers have shown promise for monitoring treatment efficacy. For example, oestrogen-containing hormone replacement therapy induces a rapid decrease in bone resorption markers that reaches a plateau within 3–6 months and is sustained as long as treatment is continued (Figure 5.8). Treatment with bisphosphonate drugs has a similar effect, although the pattern differs slightly depending on drug potency and route of administration.

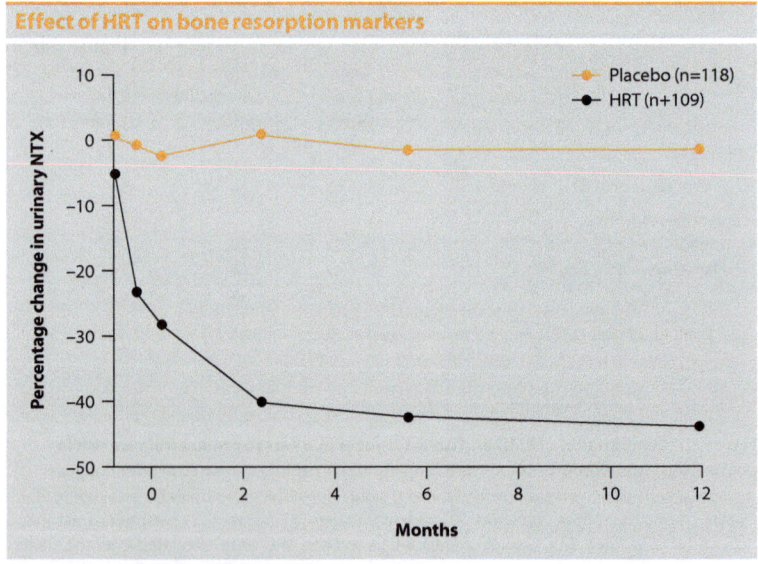

Figure 5.8 Effect of HRT on bone resorption markers. The sustained increased NTX in the placebo group was associated with bone loss. In the HRT group, NTX decreased within 2 weeks of treatment, reaching a plateau after 3 months, and was associated with increased spinal BMD. BMD, bone mineral density; HRT, hormone replacement therapy; NTX, urinary N-telopeptide of type I collagen. Data from Chesnut et al. [11].

These observations suggest that changes in biochemical markers could be used to predict the longer term response to therapy. This could potentially allow treatment to be targeted to the subset of patients who are most likely to benefit, thereby improving the cost-effectiveness of osteoporosis therapy [12]. That said, it should be remembered that the underlying principle regarding the use of BMD or biochemical markers for monitoring is that of 'least significant change' whereby, to conclude that treatment has been effective, the biochemical marker must change by more than the 95% confidence interval of the reproducibility of the technique [13].

WHO Fracture Risk Assessment Tool (FRAX)

The 10-year probability of hip and major osteoporotic fracture in men and women aged between 40 and 90 years can be estimated using the World Health Organization (WHO) Fracture Risk Assessment Tool (FRAX) [14,15]. This is primarily an online tool (available at http://www.shef.ac.uk/FRAX), although simplified paper versions are available for download. FRAX has been developed using population data from several countries including China, France, Italy, Japan, Spain, Sweden, the UK and the USA, and risk calculations are based upon entering data on known risk factors for fracture (Figure 5.9).

Kanis et al. [14] have recently used the FRAX tool to estimate the 10-year fracture risk of hip or major osteoporotic fracture in UK men and women with or without the incorporation of BMD data. Each of the clinical risk factors was separately found to influence fracture risk, with their integration into the FRAX model proved allowing prediction of the 10-year risk (Figure 5.10).

WHO Fracture Risk Assessment Tool (FRAX)

- Assesses 10-year fracture risk
- Based on input of risk factors (age, sex, height, weight, previous fracture, smoking history, glucocorticoid use, presence of rheumatoid arthritis or secondary osteoporosis, alcohol intake) and, if available, BMD
- Versions available for several countries: China, France, Italy, Japan, Spain, Sweden, UK and USA
- Available at http://www.shef.ac.uk/FRAX

Figure 5.9 WHO Fracture Risk Assessment Tool (FRAX).

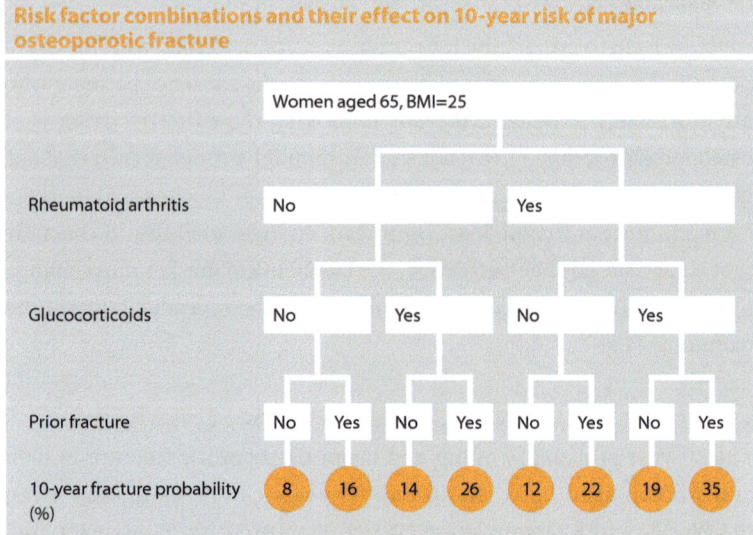

Risk factor combinations and their effect on 10-year risk of major osteoporotic fracture

Women aged 65, BMI=25

	Rheumatoid arthritis			

Figure 5.10 Risk factor combinations and their effect on 10-year risk of major osteoporotic fracture. BMI, body mass index. Reproduced with permission from Kanis JA, Johnell O, Oden A, Johansson H, McCloskey E. FRAX™ and the assessment of fracture probability in men and women from the UK. Osteoporos Int 2008;19:385–97.

Recently the 10-year risk of major osteoporotic fracture has been incorporated in a new UK-based guideline produced by the National Osteoporosis Guideline Group (NOGG). The guideline, available online at www.shef.ac.uk/NOGG, takes the output from the UK FRAX tool and determines whether treatment is indicated on cost-effectiveness grounds. Where BMD has not been included in the FRAX calculation, NOGG also determines whether BMD should be assessed to improve risk stratification [16].

References

1   North American Menopause Society. Management of postmenopausal osteoporosis: position statement of the North American Menopause Society. Menopause 2002;9:84–101.
2   Marshall D, Johnell O, Wedel H. Meta-analysis of how well measures of bone mineral density predict occurrence of osteoporotic fractures. BMJ 1996;312:1254–9.
3   Kanis JA. Diagnosis of osteoporosis and assessment of fracture risk. Lancet 2002;359:1929–36.
4   Cummings SR, Bates D, Black DM. Clinical use of bone densitometry: scientific review. JAMA 2002;288:1889–97.
5   Kanis JA, Johnell O, Oden A, et al. Ten year probabilities of osteoporotic fractures according to BMD and diagnostic thresholds. Osteoporos Int 2001;12:989–95.

6 World Health Organization (WHO). Assessment of fracture risk and its application to screening for postmenopausal osteoporosis. WHO Technical Report Series 843. Geneva: WHO, 1994.

7 Delmas PD, Eastell R, Garnero P, et al. The use of biochemical markers of bone turnover in osteoporosis. Committee of Scientific Advisors of the International Osteoporosis Foundation. Osteoporos Int 2000;11 (suppl 6):S2–17.

8 Riis BJ, Hansen MA, Jensen AM, et al. Low bone mass and fast rate of bone loss at menopause: equal risk factors for future fracture: a 15-year follow-up study. Bone 1996;19:9–12.

9 Garnero P, Hausherr E, Chapuy MC, et al. Markers of bone resorption predict hip fracture in elderly women: the EPIDOS Prospective Study. J Bone Miner Res 1996;11:1531–8.

10 Garnero P, Sornay-Rendu E, Claustrat B, et al. Biochemical markers of bone turnover, endogenous hormones and the risk of fractures in postmenopausal women: the OFELY study. J. Bone Miner Res 2000;15:1526–36.

11 Chesnut CH, Bell NH, Clark GS, et al. Hormone replacement therapy in postmenopausal women: urinary N-telopeptide of type I collagen monitors therapeutic effect and predicts response of bone mineral density. Am J Med 1997;102:29–37.

12 Schousboe JT, Bauer DC, Nyman JA, et al. Potential for bone turnover markers to cost-effectively identify and select post-menopausal osteopenic women at high risk of fracture for bisphosphonate therapy. Osteoporos Int 2007;18:201–10.

13 Hannon R, Eastell R. Preanalytical variability of biochemical markers of bone turnover. Osteoporos Int 2000;11(18, suppl 6):S30–44.

14 Kanis JA, Johnell O, Oden A, Johansson H, McCloskey E. FRAX™ and the assessment of fracture probability in men and women from the UK. Osteoporos Int 2008;19:385–97.

15 Watts NB, Lewiecki EM, Miller PD, Baim S. National Osteoporosis Foundation 2008 clinician's guide to prevention and treatment of osteoporosis and the World Health Organization Fracture Risk Assessment Tool (FRAX): what they mean to the bone densitometrist and bone technologist. J Clin Densitom 2008; 11:473–7.

16 Compston J, Cooper A, Cooper C, et al., on behalf of The National Osteoporosis Guideline Group. Guidelines for the diagnosis and managment of osteoporosis in postmenopausal women and men from the age of 50 in the UK. Maturitus 2009; 62:105–8.

Chapter 6

Non-pharmacological and adjunctive management

Non-pharmacological approaches to postmenopausal osteoporosis

All women should be encouraged to take steps to prevent bone loss and fractures, such as eating a balanced diet (including adequate intakes of calcium and vitamin D), participating in appropriate weight-bearing exercise, not smoking, avoiding excessive alcohol consumption, and instituting measures to prevent falls. Some of these steps, such as smoking cessation and exercise, offer health benefits beyond their effects on osteoporosis. Non-pharmacological treatments for post-menopausal osteoporosis are summarized in Figure 6.1 and reviewed in detail below.

Goals of intervention

The aim of management of is to prevent a first or subsequent fracture by slowing/preventing bone loss, maintaining bone strength and minimiz-ing skeletal trauma. Changes in lifestyle are helpful but women with a high fracture risk will often also need pharmacological intervention. In primary care, specific goals are to:

- maximize peak bone mass,
- identify patients at highest risk of fracture,
- use investigations cost-effectively,
- exclude secondary osteoporosis,
- provide lifestyle advice to all those at risk,

- provide appropriate drug treatment to those at highest risk and encourage compliance, and
- identify and manage those at increased risk of falls.

Recommendations for the management of osteoporosis differ by country. A treatment algorithm proposed by the Royal College of Physicians (UK) is shown in Figure 6.2 [1].

Lifestyle approaches to managing postmenopausal osteoporosis are discussed below; pharmacological management is reviewed in Chapter 7.

Diet and nutrition

A balanced diet is crucial for bone development and for general health. Elderly women are particularly prone to malnutrition as a result of

Non-pharmacological approaches to postmenopausal osteoporosis
Lifestyle changes
Smoking cessation
Regular physical exercise
• Improves muscle strength, balance, agility, coordination; may reduce risk of falling of serious fracture should a fall occur
• Weight-bearing exercise most beneficial (increases bone density)
• Benefits of exercise are rapidly lost following cessation of regular activity
Moderation of alcohol intake
Adherence to a balanced diet, rich in calcium and containing sufficient vitamin D
Prevention of falls or of effects of falls*
Wearing hip protectors
• Generally considered to reduce the incidence of hip fracture, but uncomfortable and impractical (leads to poor compliance)
• In a large randomized controlled trial of British women living independently and at high risk of fracture, there was no evidence of an effect of hip protectors among women
Wearing appropriate footwear at all times
Home modifications
• Improved lighting, handrails, well-fitting carpets
• Use of anchor rugs and non-skid mats
Physician-instigated measures
• Identification and treatment of any impairments/conditions may increase risk of falling (e.g. failing eyesight, hearing loss, neurological and rheumatological conditions)
• Avoidance of or dose minimization of drugs with sedative effects
• Referral for gait and balance training, if required

Figure 6.1 Non-pharmacological approaches to postmenopausal osteoporosis. *Most non-vertebral fractures result from falls, which occur with increasing frequency with age.

Treatment algorithm for osteoporosis

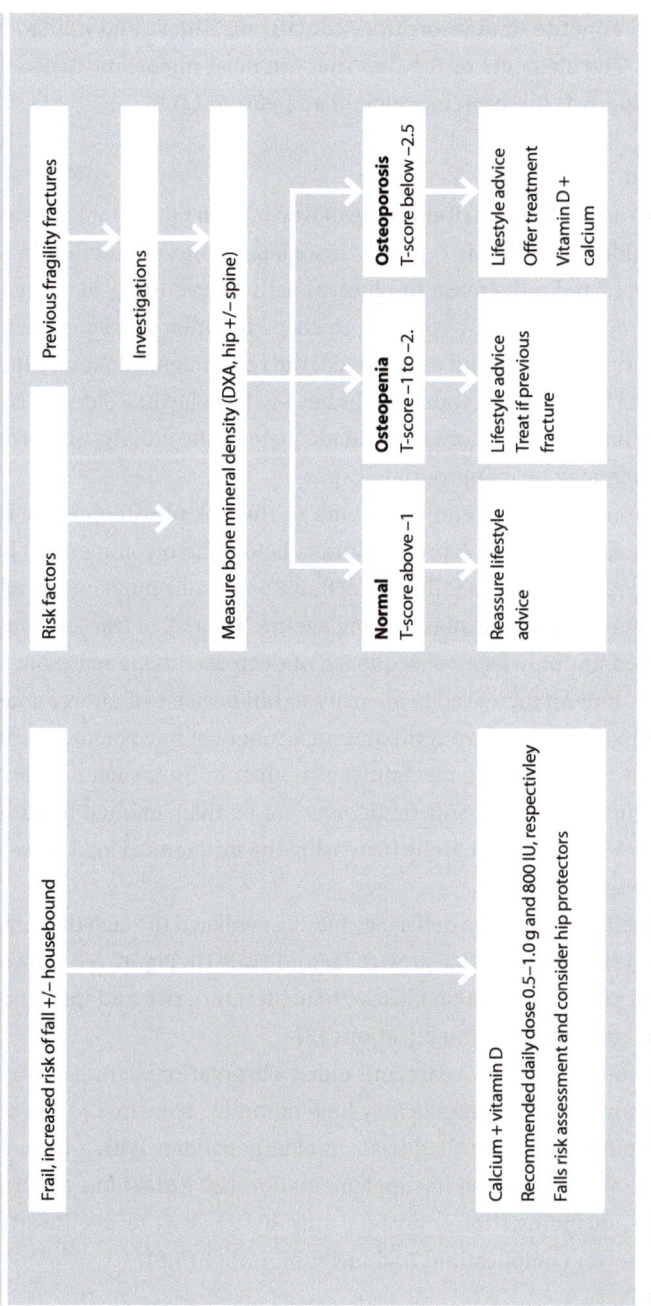

Figure 6.2 Treatment algorithm for osteoporosis. N.B. No recommendations were included in the RCP clinical guidelines regarding either strontium ranelate or teriparatide because they were not licensed when the guideline was published. DXA, dual-energy X-ray absorptiometry; HRT, hormone replacement therapy. Adapted with permission from Royal College of Physicians (RCP). Osteoporosis – Clinical guidelines for prevention and treatment. London: Royal College of Physicians, 1999.

reduced appetite, malabsorption, concurrent illness and a history of dieting. The elements of the diet that are most important to consider in osteoporosis are protein, calcium and vitamin D.

Protein

Protein–energy malnutrition is the most common nutritional deficiency in the elderly. Ageing is typically associated with a reduction in lean body mass and a decrease in physical activity, resulting in decreased energy requirements. By contrast, the need for other nutrients does not decline significantly with age. Indeed, the recommended dietary intake of protein is 0.8 g/kg in young adults but 1 g/kg in healthy elderly people. Protein intake is therefore often inadequate in the elderly, and protein restriction may be inappropriate [2].

Protein deficiency can contribute to the risk of osteoporotic fractures in various ways. A protein intake below the recommended daily allowance can result in failure to achieve peak bone mass and in a lack of preservation of bone mass during ageing. The risk of fracture may be increased not only as a consequence of decreased bone mass but also as a result of an increased propensity to fall because of altered muscle function (e.g. lack of strength) and impairment of movement coordination and the protective mechanisms against falling, such as reaction times. In addition, the soft tissue may not be thick enough to cushion the bones effectively, thereby increasing the mechanical load placed on the osteoporotic bones.

The effects of protein deficiency may be mediated through the somatomedin system [insulin-like growth factor-I (IGF-1)]. Figure 6.3 shows the possible effects of IGF-I on muscle, bone, fracture risk and incidence of post-fracture medical complications [3].

In women aged 75 years and older, observational studies suggest that adequate protein intake may help minimize bone loss [4]. In addition, randomized controlled trials in elderly patients with a recent hip fracture show that protein supplementation (20 g/day) has a range of benefits, including shorter hospital stay, better short-term clinical outcomes, fewer complications and lower mortality [5,6].

Calcium

Calcium is absorbed in the duodenum by an active mechanism regulated by 1,25-dihydroxycholecalciferol and also passively in the distal bowel. The efficiency of absorption declines with age, so calcium intake must rise in order to avoid deficiency. A number of agencies have published recommendations for dietary calcium intake at different ages. These vary widely from country to country; the current European and US recommendations are shown in Figures 6.4 and 6.5, respectively.

More than 20 randomized controlled trials have examined the impact of calcium intake on postmenopausal osteoporosis. Most of these have found that calcium supplementation is associated with an increase in BMD of around 1%. The increase in BMD is usually significant at one or more skeletal sites, and the benefits of calcium supplementation appear to be more marked in late postmenopausal life than at the perimenopause [9].

A number of studies have suggested that the impact of calcium supplementation on BMD is greatest in the first year of treatment, and occurs particularly at sites where cancellous bone predominates. There

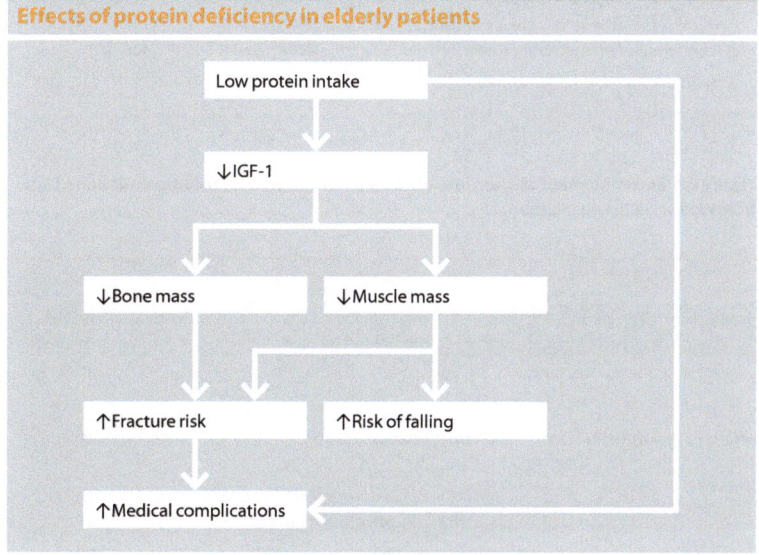

Figure 6.3 Effects of protein deficiency in elderly patients. Reproduced with permission from Rizzoli R. Atlas of Postmenopausal Osteoporosis, 2nd edition. London: Current Medicine Group Limited, 2005.

is a residual effect on BMD of around 0.25% per year after the first year, which would give a cumulative benefit of around 7.5% if the effect was sustained over 30 years [10].

A recent meta-analysis of randomized controlled trials reporting fracture rates found that calcium supplementation was associated with a relative risk (RR) of 0.77 for vertebral fracture and 0.86 for non-vertebral fracture [11]. Separately, a large international case–control study found that hip fractures were less frequent in those receiving calcium supplements (RR 0.75) [12].

Dietary sources should be the primary source of calcium intake because calcium-rich foods contain other essential nutrients; the calcium content of some common foods is shown in Figure 6.6. Supplements

Recommended calcium intake – European Community recommendations	
	Intake (mg/day)
Adults (both sexes)	
Population reference intake (intake sufficient for practically all healthy people in a population)	700
Average requirements	550
Lowest threshold limit (intake below which almost all individuals are unlikely to maintain metabolic integrity according to criterion chosen)	400
Females	
Pregnant	700
Lactating	1200

Figure 6.4 Recommended calcium intake – European Community recommendations. Data from World Health Organization [2].

Recommended calcium intake – US recommendations		
	Age group (years)	Intake (mg/day)
National Academy of Sciences	31–50	1000
	≥51	1200
National Institutes of Health	Premenopausal, 25–50	1000
	Postmenopausal:	
	<65, Using oestrogen replacement therapy	1000
	Not using oestrogen replacement therapy	1500
	All women >65	1500

Figure 6.5 Recommended calcium intake – US recommendations. Data from Institute of Medicine Standing Committee on the Scientific Evaluation of Dietary Reference Intakes [7], and National Institutes of Health, NIH Consensus Development Panel on Optimal Calcium Intake, [8].

and fortified foods are an alternative source for women who not able to consume enough dietary calcium: many women need an additional 400–800 mg/day over their daily dietary intake to reach the recommended levels, especially if they require therapy for fracture prevention. Calcium supplements are generally well tolerated, with no serious side effects. However, calcium intake greater than 2500 mg/day can increase the risk of hypercalciuria and possibly hypercalcaemia [13].

Calcium content of some common foods

Food	Calcium content(mg/100 g)	Calcium per serving (mg)
Whole milk:		
Cow	120	280
Goat	150	360
Skim milk	130	300
Yohurt	130	260
Ice cream	140	100
Cheese:		
Hard	600–1000	150–250
Soft	300–400	80–100
Cottage cheese	60	15
Broccoli, cabbage	80	80
Cauliflower, lettuce	20	10
Small fish (e.g. sardines, including bones)	460	280
Nuts (cashews/almonds)	40–250	260
Tofu	105	
Bread:		
European	30–40	10
Arabic	60–90	15–20
Vine leaves	390	18
Rice	9	96
Semolina	48	–
Seeds:		
Sesame	1200	–
Watermelon	50	–
Pine	14	–

Figure 6.6 Calcium content of some common foods. Reproduced with permission from World Health Organization (WHO). Prevention and Management of Osteoporosis. Report of a WHO Scientific Group. WHO Technical Report Series 921. Geneva: WHO, 2003.

No single laboratory test can accurately detect calcium deficiency. In general, postmenopausal women in Europe and North America have suboptimal dietary calcium intakes. Specific populations of postmenopausal women at risk of inadequate calcium intake include women who are elderly, lactose-intolerant, or vegetarian [13].

Vitamin D

Vitamin D_3 (cholecalciferol) is produced in the skin as a result of the action of ultraviolet light; the efficiency of this process is reduced with age and skin pigmentation. Indeed, vitamin D deficiency is common in the elderly, mainly because of reduced exposure to sunlight. Vitamin D is essential for the intestinal absorption of calcium, and ensuring sufficient vitamin D intake is fundamental to the prevention and treatment of osteoporosis. In relation to bone health, it does not only have a role in calcium absorption: vitamin D deficiency also leads to secondary hyperparathyroidism and consequently to greater bone loss. Deficiency also impairs muscle metabolism and may increase the likelihood of falls [2].

The recommended dietary intake of vitamin D in the USA is 400 IU/ day in women aged 51–70 years and 600 IU/day for women older than 70 years [7]. In the UK there is no recommended dietary intake for healthy young adults, but above the age of 65 there is a 4-fold decrease in the capacity of the skin to produce vitamin D. and in this age-group the recommended daily intake is 10mg [14]. Others at greatest risk of vitamin D deficiency are those with reduced sunlight exposure, such as the chronically ill, the housebound, and institutionalized women, or those who live in northern latitudes.

Dietary sources of vitamin D include fortified dairy products, fatty fish and supplements. Daily requirements can usually be met with a supplement (typically containing 400 IU vitamin D) and moderate sun exposure. The safe upper limit of vitamin D is 2000 IU/day; higher doses are associated with hypercalciuria and hypercalcaemia and should be avoided [13].

A meta-analysis of 17 randomized controlled trials confirmed the efficacy of vitamin D metabolites in improving BMD and reducing fractures. All patients had established osteoporosis and some had been exposed to corticosteroids. Overall, the use of vitamin D metabolites (namely, alphacalcidol and calcitriol) significantly reduced the risk of vertebral and non-vertebral fracture, and improved BMD, regardless of whether or not the vitamin D was given along with calcium.

Some randomized controlled trials have found that co-administration of calcium and native vitamin D reduces fracture risk in elderly individuals. In one study involving 3000 elderly women, vitamin D 800 IU and calcium 1200 mg daily reduced the risk of non-vertebral and hip fractures by one-quarter (RR 0.75) (Figure 6.7) [15]. Another study in 400 men and women aged 65 years and over found that daily supplementation

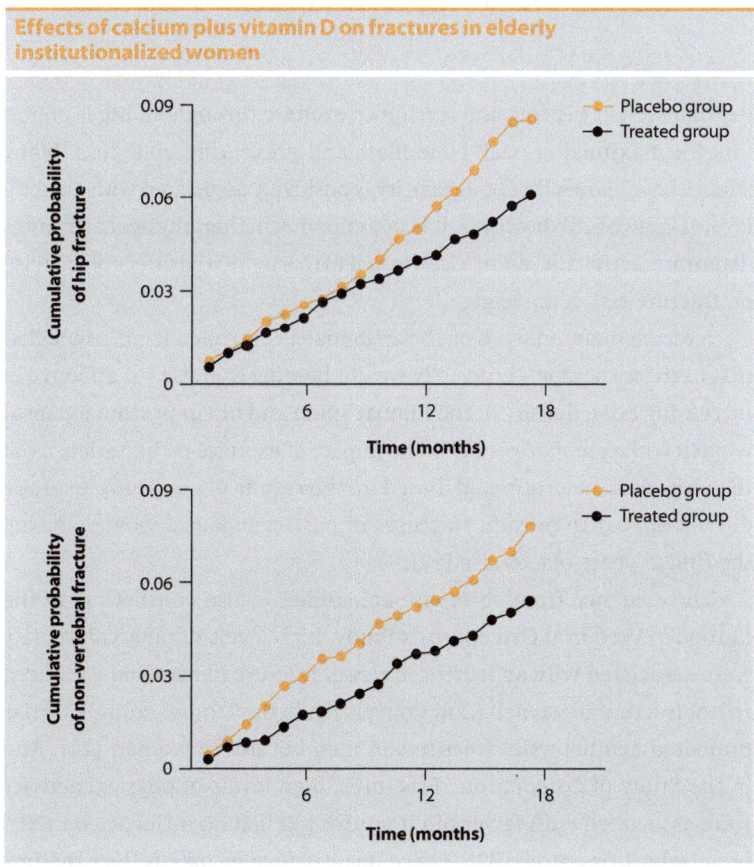

Effects of calcium plus vitamin D on fractures in elderly institutionalized women

Figure 6.7 Effects of calcium plus vitamin D on fractures in elderly institutionalized women.
Data from Chapuy MC, Arlot ME, Duboeuf F, et al. Vitamin D3 and calcium to prevent hip fractures in the elderly women. N Engl J Med 1992;327:1637-42.

with calcium 500 mg plus vitamin D 700 IU reduced non-vertebral fracture rates by more than one-half (RR 0.45) [16]. However the routine use of calcium and vitamin D in healthy 'free-living' elderly has been cast in doubt by the publication of more recent RCTs which have shown no effect. The largest of these carried out in the UK (The RECORD trial) showed no difference in fracture rates in those who had already sustained a low-trauma fracture and who were supplemented with calcium, calcium and vitamin D, vitamin D alone or placebo [17].

Recent interest has focused on the role of vitamin D in protecting against falls, which has been demonstrated in a recent meta-analysis [18].

Exercise

Regular weight-bearing and resistance exercise throughout life is important for maximizing peak bone mass and preventing bone loss. Many studies have shown that bone density is positively associated with exercise levels (Figure 6.8); however, it is not known whether physical attributes determine activity levels or vice versa. Furthermore, the effect of exercise on fracture risk is unclear.

A recent meta-analysis of 18 randomized controlled trials concluded that exercise therapy – especially weight-bearing exercise – is effective in increasing bone density at the lumbar spine and hip in postmenopausal women with osteoporosis [19]. The impact of exercise on bone density at the wrist was uncertain and, based on the results of one study, exercise did not appear to prevent fractures in postmenopausal women during the first 2 years of exercise [19].

The evidence from observational studies is also conflicting. In the European Vertebral Osteoporosis Study, high levels of physical activity were associated with an increased risk of fracture in men and a reduced risk of fracture in women [20]. Conversely, in the Tromsø study, exercise protected against axial fractures in men but not in women [21]. And in the Study of Osteoporotic Fractures, high levels of physical activity were associated with fewer hip fractures but had no influence on wrist or vertebral fractures [22]. These inconsistencies may reflect the fact that exercise is associated not only with increased bone density but also with increased exposure to skeletal trauma.

The principal contribution of exercise in women with postmenopausal osteoporosis is probably to maintain muscle strength and thus prevent falls. Women should be encouraged to participate in exercise programs that include training for balance, but they should not perform heavy weight-bearing exercise or activities vigorous enough to trigger a fracture. Individually tailoured exercise programmes that include Tai Chi may be valuable but have not been shown to improve BMD [23].

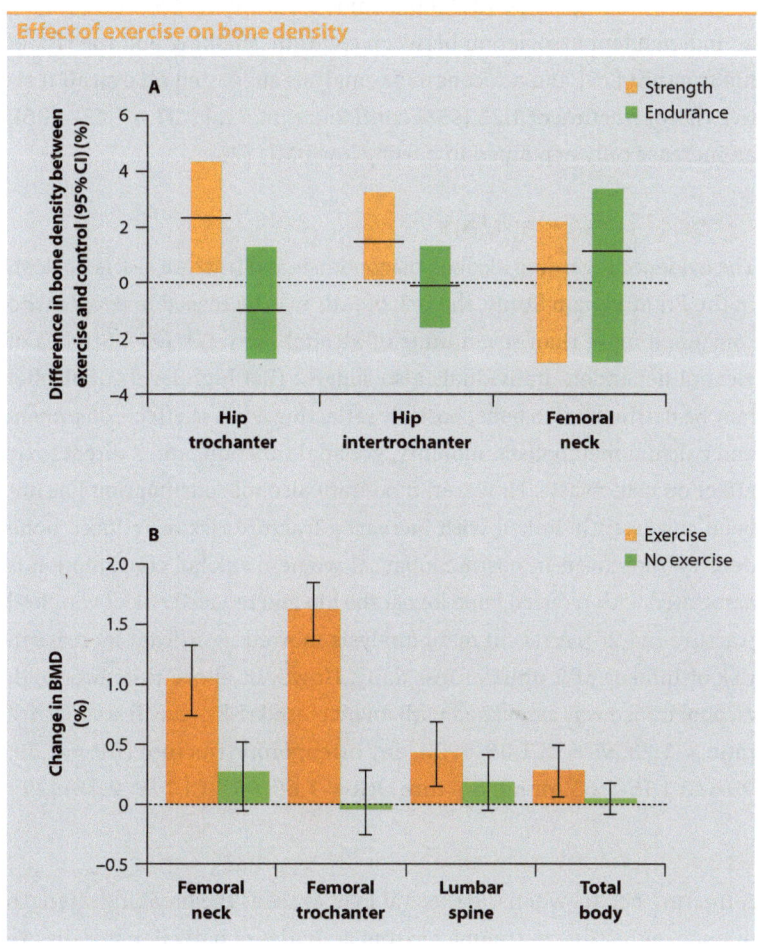

Effect of exercise on bone density

Figure 6.8 Effect of exercise on bone density. Adapted with permission from Going S, Lohman T, Houtkooper L, et al. Effects of exercise on bone mineral density in calcium-replete postmenopausal women with and without hormone replacement therapy. Osteoporos Int 2003; 14:637–43.

Smoking cessation

Women should be encouraged to cease smoking because it lowers BMD through a number of mechanisms, including reduced peak bone mass, earlier menopause, reduced body weight, and enhanced metabolic breakdown of exogenous oestrogen [24]. A meta-analysis of 48 studies found that bone density in women smokers fell by around 2% per decade after the age of 50 years, leading to a 6% difference between smokers and non-smokers at the age of 80 [25]. Epidemiological studies have also shown an independent association between cigarette smoking and the risk of hip fracture [25] and a recent meta-analysis suggested an overall relative risk of fracture of 1.25 [95% confidence interval (CI) = 1.15–1.36], an increase only explained in part by low BMD [26].

Alcohol consumption

The evidence regarding alcohol, osteoporosis and fracture risk is unclear. In the Framingham Study, the risk of falls was increased in people who consumed more than seven units of alcohol per week [27]. Studies of alcohol-dependent individuals also suggest that high levels of alcohol may be detrimental to bone, possibly reflecting adverse effects on protein and calcium metabolism, mobility, gonadal function, and a direct toxic effect on osteoblasts. However, moderate alcohol consumption has not been consistently linked with increased fracture risk or reduced bone density. Moreover, in postmenopausal women, alcohol consumption is associated with reduced bone loss at the hip and reduced risk of vertebral fracture [24,28]. A recent meta-analysis showed significant increase in risk at intakes of 2 units or less daily. However, above this threshold, alcohol intake was associated with an increased risk of any fracture (risk ratio = 1.23; 95% CI 1.06–1.43), any osteoporotic fracture (RR = 1.38; 95% CI 1.16–1.65) or hip fracture (RR = 1.68; 95% CI 1.19–2.36) [29].

Prevention of and protection against falls

A fracture occurs when the skeletal load exceeds the breaking strength of bone, either due to trauma or from activities of daily living. Falls are the most common cause of traumatic osteoporotic fractures. Fortunately, however, only a minority of falls lead to a fracture. The likelihood of a fracture depends on many factors, including the orientation of the fall, the person's body weight, the amount of soft tissue over the bone, and the bone density [30]. Risk factors associated with hip fracture after a fall are shown in Figure 6.9.

The annual risk of falling increases with age, from around 20% in women aged 35–59 years to 50% in women aged 80 years and over [31]. Elderly women have a significantly higher risk for falls than do men of the same age; similarly, people living in nursing and residential homes are around three times more likely to fall than their counterparts living in the community.

Women with postmenopausal osteoporosis should be assessed for the risk of falls. Risk assessment should cover clinical factors, such as a history of falls, fainting, or loss of consciousness; muscle weakness, dizziness, or balance problems; problems with neuromuscular coordination; and impaired vision. Other considerations include chronic illness, such as neurological disorders, stroke, urinary incontinence, depression, and impaired cognitive function, and medications that affect balance and coordination, such as hypnotics, narcotic analgesics, anticholinergics, and sedatives. Environmental hazards play a role in many falls: potential dangers in the home include obstacles, poor lighting, slippery floors, and unstable furniture [32].

Many of the risk factors for falling are modifiable, for example, by correcting eye problems and installing adequate lighting. Multifactorial interventions that can help reduce the risk of falls when targeted at high-risk individuals are summarized in Figure 6.10.

Risk factors associated with hip fracture from a fall	
Factor	**Adjusted odds ratio (95% CI)**
Direct hip impact	4.9 (2.7–8.8)
Previous stroke	2.9 (1.3–6.3)
Sideways fall	2.5 (1.6–3.9)
Functional mobility	2.0 (1.1–3.5)
Body mass index	1.8 (1.1–2.8)
Femoral neck bone mineral density	1.7 (1.0–2.8)

Figure 6.9 Risk factors associated with hip fracture from a fall. Adapted with permission from Wei TS, Hu CH, Wang SH, et al. Fall characteristics, functional mobility and bone mineral density as risk factors of hip fracture in the community-dwelling ambulatory elderly. Osteoporos Int 2001; 12:1050–5.

People at high risk of fracture may also be advised to wear energy-absorbing hip protectors to minimize the impact of falls should they occur (Figure 6.11). However, compliance may be poor, the devices are expensive, and their efficacy in preventing hip fracture has not been established [33–35]. Hip protectors are likely to be acceptable only to women living in nursing or residential homes, and even in this group compliance and hygiene are a problem.

Interventions to decrease risk of falls

- Medication assessment
- Intervention for postural hypotension
- Environment hazard modification
- Gain training and advice on use of walking sticks and Zimmer frames
- Exercise programmes including balance training and Tai Chi
- Treatment of comorbid cardiovascular problems

Figure 6.10 Interventions to decrease risk of falls.

Hip protectors

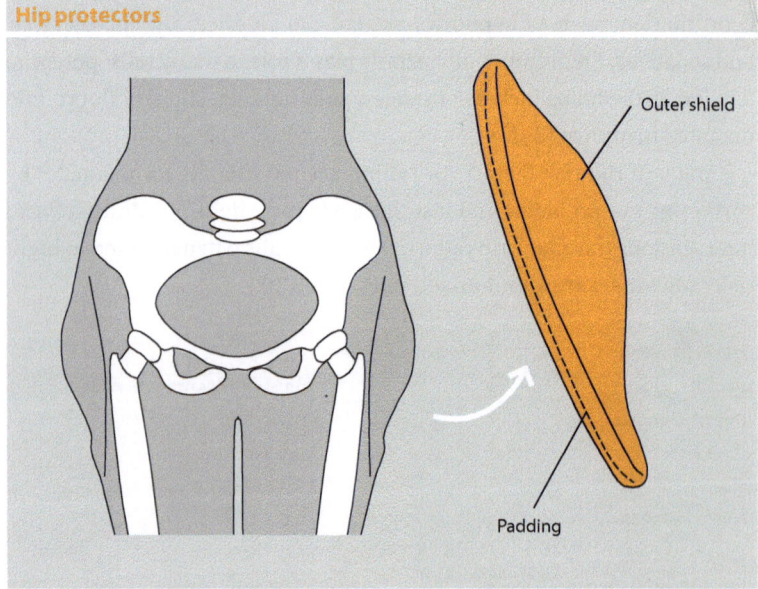

Outer shield

Padding

Figure 6.11 Hip protectors. Reproduced with permission from Kannus P, Pakkaris J, Niemi S, et al. Prevention of hip fracture in elderly people with use of a hip protector. N Engl J Med 2000; 343:1506–13.

References

1 Royal College of Physicians. Osteoporosis: clinical guidelines for prevention and treatment. London: Royal College of Physicians; 1999.

2 World Health Organization (WHO). Prevention and management of osteoporosis. report of a WHO scientific group. WHO Technical Report Series 921. Geneva: WHO, 2003.

3 Rizzoli R, Ammann P, Chevalley T, et al. Protein intake and bone disorders in the elderly. Joint Bone Spine 2001;68:383–92.

4 Hannan MT, Tucker KL, Dawson-Hughes B, et al. Effect of dietary protein on bone loss in elderly men and women: the Framingham Osteoporosis Study. J Bone Miner Res 2000;15:2504–12.

5 Delmi M, Rapin CH, Bengoa JM,et al. Dietary supplementation in elderly patients with fractured neck of the femur. Lancet 1990;335:1013–1016.

6 Tkatch L, Rapin CH, Rizzoli R, et al. Benefits of oral protein supplementation in elderly patients with fracture of the proximal femur. J Am Coll Nutr 1992;11:519–25.

7 Institute of Medicine. Standing Committee on the Scientific Evaluation of Dietary Reference Intakes. Dietary reference intakes: calcium, phosphorus, magnesium, vitamin D, and fluoride. Washington, DC: National Academy Press, 1997.

8 National Institutes of Health. NIH Consensus Development Panel on Optimal Calcium Intake. Optimal calcium intake. JAMA 1994;272:1942–8.

9 Nordin BEC. Calcium and osteoporosis. Nutrition 1997;13:664–86.

10 Reid IR, Ames RW, Evans MC, et al. Long-term effects of calcium supplementation on bone loss and fractures in postmenopausal women – a randomized controlled trial. Am J Med 1995;98:331–335.

11 Shea B, Wells G, Cranney A, et al. Meta-analyses of therapies for postmenopausal osteoporosis. VII. Meta-analysis of calcium supplementation for the prevention of postmenopausal osteoporosis. Endocrine Rev 2002;23:552–9.

12 Kanis JA, Johnell O, Gullberg B, et al. Evidence for efficacy of drugs affecting bone metabolism in preventing hip fracture. BMJ 1992;305:1124–8.

13 North American Menopause Society. Management of postmenopausal osteoporosis: position statement of the North American Menopause Society. Menopause 2002;9:84–101.

14 Department of Health. Nutrition and bone health: with particular reference to calcium and vitamin D. London, The London Stationery Office, 1998.

15 Chapuy MC, Arlot ME, Delmas PD, et al. Effect of calcium and cholecalciferol treatment for three years on hip fractures in elderly women. BMJ 1994;308:1081–82.

16 Dawson-Hughes B, Harris SS, Krall EA, et al. Effect of calcium and vitamin D supplementation on bone, density in men and women 65 years of age or older. N Engl J Med 1997;337:670–676.

17 Grant AM, Avenell A, Campbell MK et al. Oral vitamin D_3 and calcium for secondary prevention of low-trauma fractures in elderly people (Randomised Evaluation of Calcium Or vitamin D, RECORD): a randomised placebo-controlled trial. Lancet 2005;365:1621–8

18 Bischoff-Ferrari HA, Dawson-Hughes B, Willett WC, et al. Effect of vitamin D on falls: a meta-analysis. JAMA 2004;291:1999–2006.

19 Bonaiuti D, Shea B, Iovine R, et al. Exercise for preventing and treating osteoporosis in postmenopausal women. Cochrane Database Syst Rev 2002;3:CD000333.

20 Silman AJ, O'Neill TW, Cooper C, et al. Influence of physical activity on vertebral deformity in men and women – results from the European Vertebral Osteoporosis Study. J Bone Miner Res 1997;12:813–19.

21 Joakimsen RM, Fønnebø V, Magnus JH, et al. The Tromsø study – physical activity and the incidence of fractures in a middle-aged population. J Bone Miner Res 1998;13:1149–57.

22 Gregg EW, Cauley JA, Seeley DG, et al. Physical activity and osteoporotic fracture risk in older women. Ann Intern Med 1998;129:81–8.

23 Lee MS, Pittler MH, Shin BC, Ernst E. Tai chi for osteoporosis: a systematic review. Osteoporosis Int 2008;19:139–46.

24 Seeman E. The effects of tobacco and alcohol use on bone. In: Marcus R, Feldman D, Kelsey J, eds. Osteoporosis. San Diego: Academic Press, 1996:577–97.

25 Law MR, Hackshaw AK. A meta-analysis of cigarette smoking, bone mineral density and risk of hip fracture: recognition of a major effect. BMJ 1997;315:841–6.

26 Kanis JA, Johnell O, Oden A, Johansson H, et al. Smoking and fracture risk: a meta-analysis. Osteoporos Int 2005;16:155–62.

27 Cummings SR. Epidemiology of hip fractures. In: Christiansen C, Johansen JS, Riis BJ, eds. Osteoporosis. Viborg: Norhaven A/S, 1987:40–43.

28 Naves-Diaz M, O'Neill TW, Silman A. The influence of alcohol consumption on the risk of vertebral deformity. The European Vertebral Osteoporosis Study Group. Osteoporos Int 1997;7:65–71.

29 Kanis JA, Johansson H, Johnell O, et al. Alcohol intake as a risk factor for fracture. Osteoporos Int 2005;16:737–42.

30 Greenspan SL, Myers ER, Maitland LA, et al. Fall severity and bone mineral density as risk factors for hip fracture in ambulatory elderly. JAMA 1994;271:128–33.

31 Winner SJ, Morgan CA, Evans JG. Perimenopausal risk of falling and incidence of distal forearm fracture. BMJ 1989;298:1486–8.

32 Grisso JA, Capezuti E, Schwartz A. Falls as risk factors for fractures. In: Marcus R, Feldman D, Kelsey J eds. Osteoporosis. San Diego: Academic Press, 1996:599–611.

33 Patel S, Ogunremi L, Chinappen U. Acceptability and compliance with hip protectors in community-dwelling women at high risk of hip fracture. Rheumatol 2003;42:769–72.

34 van Schoor N, Smit J, Twisk J, et al. Prevention of hip fractures by external hip protectors: a randomized controlled trial. JAMA 2003;289:1957–62.

35 Colon-Emeric CS, Lyles KW, House P, et al. Randomized trial to improve fracture prevention in nursing home residents. Am J Med 2007;120:886–92.

Chapter 7

Pharmacological treatment

Pharmacological treatment is indicated for women with postmenopausal osteoporosis or borderline bone mineral density (BMD) measurements in the presence of additional risk factors, and for women for whom non-pharmacological approaches have failed to prevent further bone loss or low-impact fractures. The availability of the new FRAX tool (see Chapter 5) has enabled intervention thresholds to be developed based on 10-year fracture prediction. In the USA universal thresholds for intervention have been suggested by the National Osteoporosis Foundation based on those who have a >20% 10-year risk of major osteoporotic fracture or a >3% risk of hip fracture [1]. In the UK a consensus group has recently launched national guidelines showing a cost-effective but variable threshold for intervention based on FRAX output but taking into account the steep rise of risk with age [2].

Therapies for osteoporosis tend to be classified as antiresorptive or anabolic (bone-forming) agents. Antiresorptive agents include:

- bisphosphonates,
- oestrogens,
- selective oestrogen receptor modulators (SERMs),
- calcitonin, and
- calcium plus vitamin D.

Calcium and vitamin D are considered to be adjunctive therapy (see Chapter 6) rather than therapeutic options to be used alone.

The evidence for the efficacy of many of the various antiresorptive therapies is summarized in Figure 7.1. Synthetic parathyroid hormone extracts are the only true anabolic agents currently marketed. Both recombinant 1–84 (PTH) and 1–34 (teriparatide) amino acid versions are available. Strontium ranelate is the first in a new class of drugs that has simultaneous antiresorptive and anabolic properties, at least in animal studies. Denosumab is another new agent that specifically targets RANKL, which is an essential mediator in osteoclast formation, function and survival (see Chapter 2). Each of these pharmacological treatment options is reviewed in detail below.

Bisphosphonates

Bisphosphonates are a class of potent antiresorptive drugs that are indicated as first-line therapy for the prevention and treatment of post-menopausal osteoporosis. Some bisphosphonates are also indicated for the treatment of glucocorticoid-induced and male osteoporosis.

Evidence for the efficacy of antiresorptive therapies in osteoporosis

Intervention	BMD	Vertebral fracture	Non-vertebral fracture	Hip fracture
Calcium	A	B	B	D
Calcium + vitamin D	–	A	A	
Oestrogens	A	A	A	A
Tibolone	A	–	–	–
Alendronate	A	A	A	A
Etidronate	A	B	D	D
Risedronate	A	A	A	A
Ibandronate	A	–	–	–
Calcitonin	A	C	C	D
Fluoride	A	C	–	–
Anabolic steroids	A	–	–	D
Calcitriol	C	C	–	D
Alfacalcidol	C	C	–	D
Raloxifene	A	A	–	–
Ipriflavone	B	–	–	–
Menatetrenone	B	B	–	–

Figure 7.1 Evidence for the efficacy of antiresorptive therapies in osteoporosis. Evidence A, positive evidence from one or more, adequately powered, randomized controlled trials; B, positive evidence from similar non-definitive randomized controlled trials; C, inconsistent results from randomized controlled trials; D, positive results from observational studies; –, efficacy not established or not tested. Reproduced with permission from World Health Organization (WHO). Prevention and management of osteoporosis. report of a who scientific group. WHO Technical Report Series 921. Geneva: WHO, 2003.

Bisphosphonates are stable synthetic analogues of pyrophosphate, an endogenous inhibitor of bone resorption (Figure 7.2). They are characterized by a phosphorous–carbon–phosphorous backbone and have a high affinity for the hydroxyapatite crystals in bone. The potency of bisphosphonates depends on the length and structure of the side chain (Figure 7.3).

The primary effect of bisphosphonates is to suppress osteoclast-mediated bone resorption (Figure 7.4). First-generation bisphosphonates (e.g. clodronate, etidronate and tiludronate) do not contain amino groups. They are metabolized to form cytotoxic ATP analogues that accumulate intracellularly in osteoclasts and induce apoptosis. Newer, nitrogen-containing bisphosphonates (e.g. alendronate, ibandronate, pamidronate, risedronate, zolendronate) interfere with the mevalonate pathway and inhibit the recruitment and function of osteoclasts (Figure 7.4).

General structure of pyrophosphate and bisphosphonates

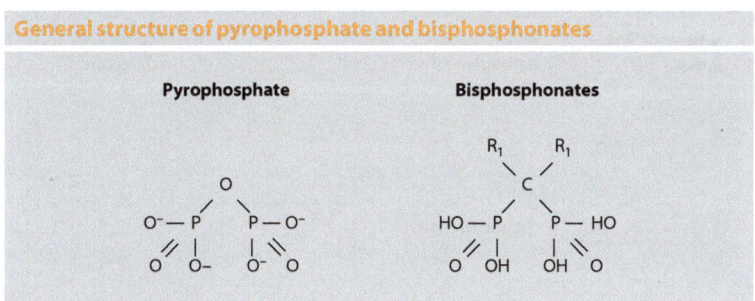

Figure 7.2 General structure of pyrophosphate and bisphosphonates.

In vitro potency of bisphosphonates

Drug	Potency
Etidronate	1
Tiludronate, clodronate	10
Pamidronate	100
Alendronate	100–1000
Risedronate	1000–10,000
Ibandronate	1000–10,000
Zolendronate	>10,000

Figure 7.3 In vitro potency of bisphosphonates. Reproduced with permission from Deal C. Osteoporosis therapies bisphosphonates, SERMs, PTH, and new therapies. Clin Rev Bone Min Metab 2005;3:125–41.

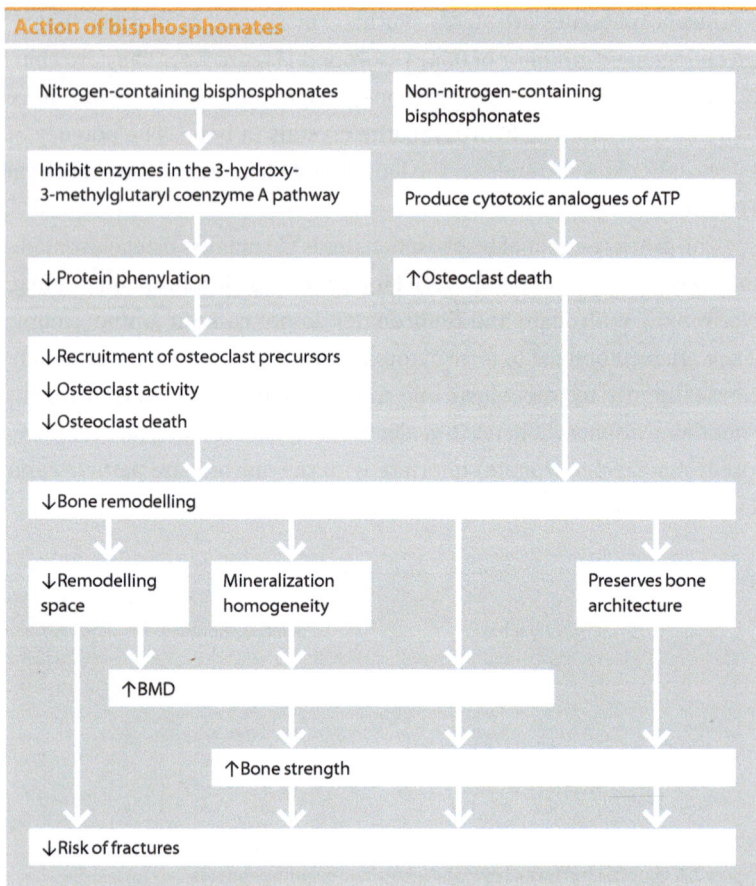

Figure 7.4 Action of bisphosphonates. ATP, Adenosine triphosphate; BMD, bone mineral density. Adapted with permission from McClung MR. Bisphosphonates. Endocrinol Metab Clin North Am 2003;32:253–71.

This section will focus on indications, dosages and trial result for the bisphosphonates that are licensed for treatment of osteoporosis. More general information on bisphosphonates as first- and second-line therapy, and on their tolerability and side effects, are given towards the end of this section. Other bisphosphonates are used solely for treatment of Paget's disease, hypercalcaemia of malignancy disease and bone metastases and so are not discussed in this book (pamidronate, clodronate and tiludronic).

Alendronate

Alendronate is a second-generation bisphosphonate that is approved for the treatment and prevention of postmenopausal osteoporosis. It has well-documented efficacy in preventing bone loss and reducing the risk of hip and vertebral fracture.

For example, the Fracture Intervention Trial (FIT), a large randomized controlled trial (RCT), included postmenopausal women with low BMD at the femoral neck, either with (FIT I, n = 2027) or without (FIT II, n = 4432) prevalent vertebral fractures [3,4]. Women were randomized to treatment with alendronate 5–10 mg/day or placebo plus supplementary calcium/vitamin D. Irrespective of the presence of prior vertebral fracture, alendronate significantly increased lumbar and hip BMD and significantly decreased the risk of vertebral fractures (Figure 7.5). However, treatment reduced the risk of hip fracture only in women with prevalent vertebral fracture and did not reduce the risk of non-vertebral fracture in either group, although wrist fractures were reduced in those with low BMD and a vertebral fracture [4].

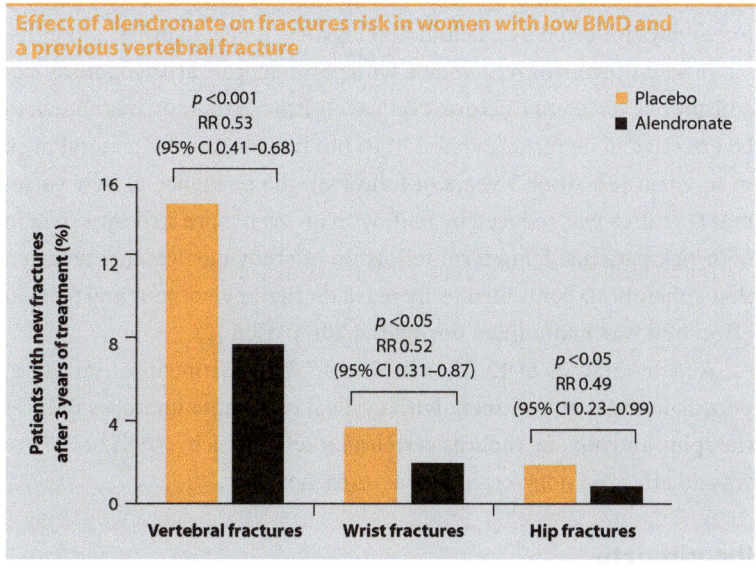

Figure 7.5 Effect of alendronate on fractures risk in women with low BMD and a previous vertebral fracture. BMD, bone mineral density; CI, Confidence interval; RR, relative risk. Data from Black et al. [4].

The efficacy of alendronate in women with postmenopausal osteo-porosis is supported by a meta-analysis of 11 RCTs [5]. At doses of 5–40 mg/day, alendronate was associated with relative risk of 0.52 for vertebral fracture and 0.51 for non-vertebral fracture. In a separate meta-analysis, which included six RCTs, alendronate 5–20 mg/day significantly reduced the risk of hip fracture, risk reduction being 0.55 [6].

Oral alendronate given once-weekly (70 mg), twice-weekly (35 mg) and daily (10 mg) has been shown to have a similar impact on BMD at the lumbar spine, femoral neck, trochanter and total hip – a site including the entire proximal femur identified on a BMD scan – and it reduced markers of bone turnover to premenopausal levels [7]. The once-weekly dosing regimen is now widely used in view of its greater convenience. A formulation of alendronate with 2800 IU vitamin D is also available.

Etidronate

Etidronate was the first bisphosphonate to be studied for use in osteo-porosis. It may impair bone mineralization when used continuously, so instead it is given in an intermittent cyclical pattern of 400 mg/day for 14 days followed by calcium 500 mg/day, repeated every 3 months.

In a RCT involving 429 women with postmenopausal osteoporosis and a history of vertebral fracture, cyclical etidronate therapy was shown to be effective in increasing spinal BMD but not BMD at the femoral neck or forearm [8]. After 3 years of follow-up the incidence of new verte-bral fractures was reduced by half, with an even more striking effect in high-risk patients. Long-term follow-up of study participants revealed that spinal BMD continued to increase on therapy without any plateau effect and was maintained during the 'off' period [9].

A meta-analysis of 13 RCTs in women with postmenopausal osteo-porosis found that treatment with cyclical etidronate improves BMD at the spine and hip and reduces vertebral fracture risk by 37% [10]. There was no effect on non-vertebral fractures, however.

Ibandronate

Ibandronate is a third-generation bisphosphonate that is approved for the prevention and treatment of postmenopausal osteoporosis. It was the first bisphosphonate to become available as an oral monthly therapy and is also available as a 3-monthly intravenous injection.

The efficacy of ibandronate in preventing fracture was established in the BONE study (oral iBandronate Osteoporosis vertebral fracture trial in North America and Europe), a RCT involving 2946 postmenopausal women with osteoporosis, a BMD T-score of –2.0 to –5.0 in at least one vertebra, and at least one vertebral fracture [11]. Study subjects were randomized to ibandronate administered daily (2.5 mg/day) or intermittently (20 mg every other day for 12 doses, repeated every 3 months). In this study, both ibandronate groups showed significant and progressive increases in BMD at the lumbar spine compared with placebo. Furthermore, the incidence of new vertebral fractures after 3 years was significantly lower in both ibandronate groups compared with placebo (Figure 7.6). Interestingly, the reduction in vertebral fracture was comparable between the daily and intermittent dosing groups, with risk reduction of 62 and 50%, respectively. This was the first time a bisphosphonate had been found effective in preventing fracture when administered intermittently with a more-than-daily dose-free interval. However no efficacy was seen in reducing non-vertebral fractures except in a small high-risk subset (T score < –3.0).

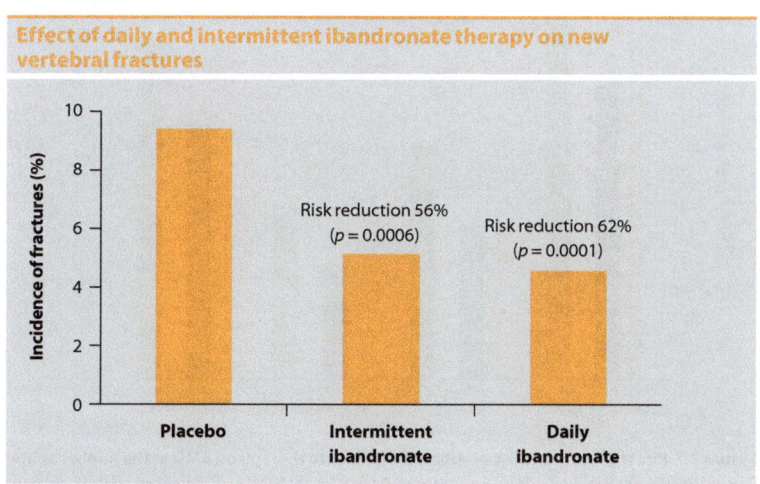

Figure 7.6 Effect of daily and intermittent ibandronate therapy on new vertebral fractures. Data from Chestnut et al. [11].

Subsequently, the therapeutic equivalence of daily and monthly ibandronate dosing was demonstrated in the MOBILE (Monthly Oral iBandronate In LadiEs) study, which included 1609 women aged 55–80 years with postmenopausal osteoporosis. They were randomized to one of four treatment regimens: 2.5 mg daily, 50+50 mg once-monthly (50 mg dose given for two consecutive days), 100 mg once-monthly and 150 once-monthly. After 2 years, BMD at the lumbar spine had increased in all four groups, with the greatest improvement occurring in the 150 mg/month group (6.6 versus 5.0% for daily dosing). Ibandronate therapy was also associated with improvements in BMD at the total hip, femoral neck and trochanter, with monthly dosing being superior to daily dosing at all sites (Figure 7.7) [12].

More recently, the DIVA (Dosing IntraVenous Administration) study demonstrated that intermittent intravenous ibandronate was at least as effective as daily oral dosing, which has established antifracture efficacy [13]. The study randomized 1395 women with postmenopausal

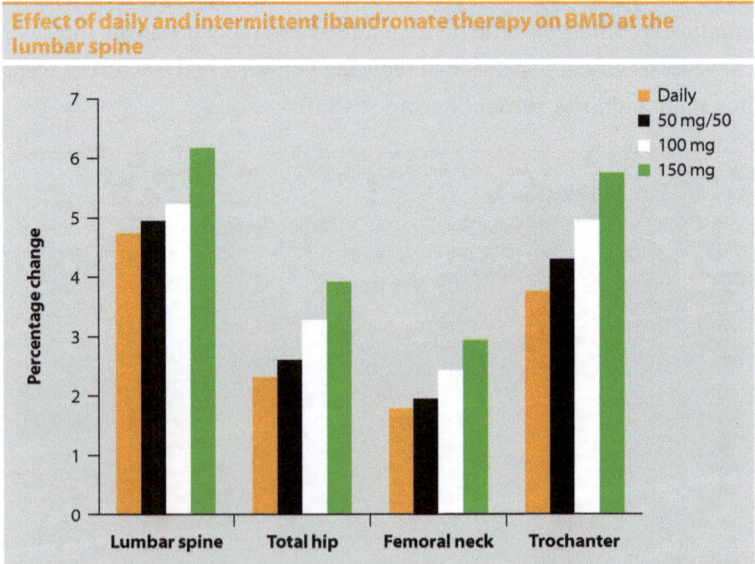

Effect of daily and intermittent ibandronate therapy on BMD at the lumbar spine

Figure 7.7 Effect of daily and intermittent ibandronate therapy on BMD at the lumbar spine. Reproduced with permission from Reginster JY, Adami S, Lakatos P, et al. Efficacy and tolerability of once-monthly oral ibandronate in postmenopausal osteoporosis: 2 year results from the MOBILE study. Ann Rheum Dis 2006;65:654–61.

osteoporosis to ibandronate given orally (2.5 mg/day) or intravenously (2 mg 2-monthly or 3 mg 3-monthly). After 1 year, BMD at the lumbar spine had risen in all three groups; the greatest increase (4.8%) occurred in the 3 mg 3-monthly group. Indeed, both intravenous regimens were found to be superior to oral dosing and were similarly well-tolerated, indicating a potential role for intravenous ibandronate in women who cannot tolerated or comply with oral therapy.

Risedronate

Risedronate is a third-generation bisphosphonate approved for the prevention and treatment of postmenopausal osteoporosis, as well as for glucocorticoid-induced osteoporosis.

The efficacy of risedronate in postmenopausal women with a prior vertebral fracture was demonstrated in the Vertebral Efficacy with Risedronate (VERT) trial, which included a North American arm (VERT-NA, n = 2458) [14] and a European/Australian arm (VERT-MN, n = 1226) [15]. After 3 years, women treated with risedronate 5 mg/day showed an increase in BMD at the lumbar spine and hips compared with the placebo group. Moreover, vertebral fractures were reduced by 41 and 49% and non-vertebral fractures were reduced by 39 and 33% in the VERT-NA and VERT-MN arms, respectively. Results from VERT-NA are shown in Figure 7.8.

Risedronate was also assessed in the Hip Intervention Program (HIP), the only trial of its kind to use hip fracture as the primary endpoint [16]. This RCT included two groups of women: those aged 70–79 years with low BMD (group 1, n = 5445) and those aged 80 and over with at least one non-skeletal risk factor for hip fracture regardless of BMD (group 2, n = 3886). Treatment was associated with 40 and 20% reductions in hip fracture incidence in groups 1 and 2, respectively (Figure 7.9); the reduction in group 2 was not statistically significant, however. Post hoc analysis of group 1 also indicated that risedronate reduced the risk of vertebral fracture by 60% compared with placebo.

Finally, a 2002 meta-analysis of eight RCTs showed that risedronate therapy was associated with a relative risk of 0.64 for vertebral fracture and 0.73 for non-vertebral fracture in postmenopausal women [17].

Effect of risedronate on incidence of new vertebral and non-vertebral fractures in VERT-NA

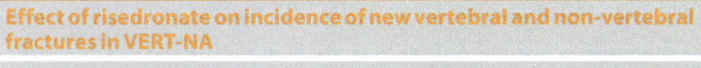

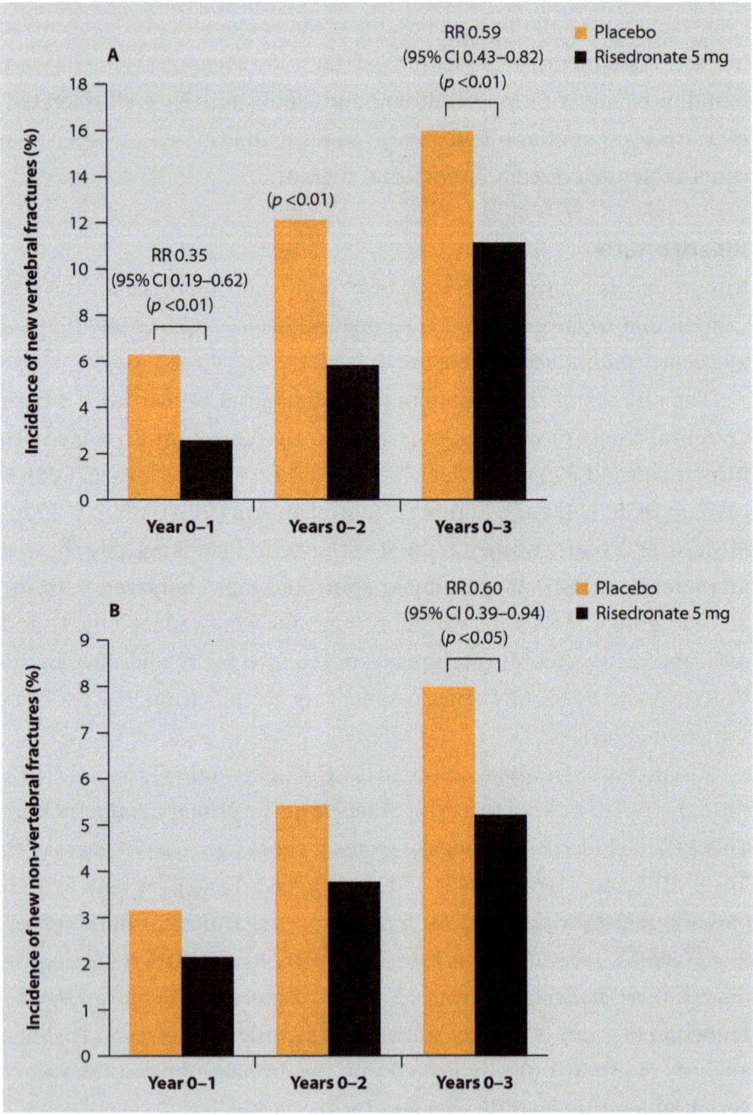

Figure 7.8 Effect of risedronate on incidence of new vertebral and non-vertebral fractures in VERT-NA. CI, Confidence interval; RR, relative risk. Adapted with permission from Harris ST, Watts NB, Genant HK et al. Effects of risedronate treatment on vertebral and nonvertebral fractures in women with postmenopausal osteoporosis. A randomized controlled trial. JAMA 1999; 282:1344–52.

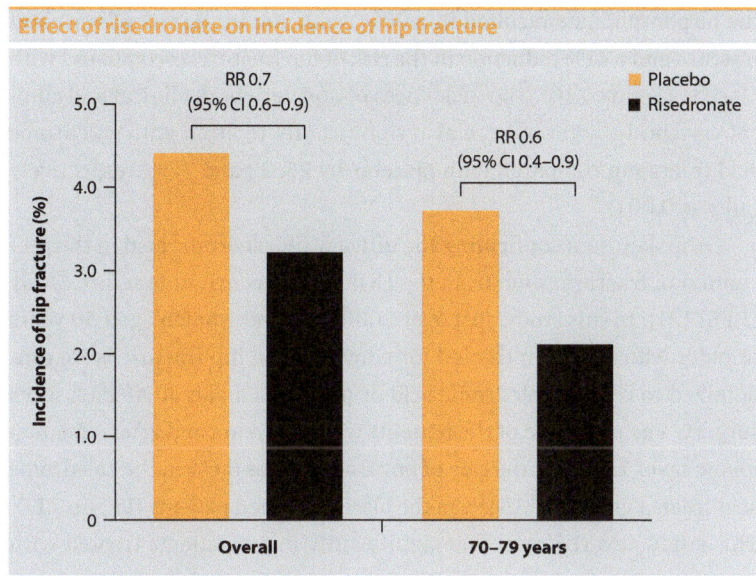

Figure 7.9 Effect of risedronate on incidence of hip fracture. CI, Confidence interval; RR, relative risk. Data from McClung et al. [16].

Zoledronic acid

Zoledronic acid is a third-generation bisphosphonate that has recently been approved as a once-yearly intravenous infusion for the prevention of osteoporotic fracture in postmenopausal women [18,19]. In clinical studies, zoledronic acid has been shown to increase BMD, decrease bone turnover markers, and be associated with a favourable adverse event profile that makes it a useful alternative to orally administered bisphosphonates.

The first trial to specifically examine the use of zoledronic acid to prevent osteoporotic fractures was the Health Outcomes and Reduced Incidence with Zoledronic Acid Once Yearly (HORIZON) Pivotal Fracture Trial (PFT) [20]. In this double blind, placebo-controlled trial, over 7000 postmenopausal women (mean age 73 years) with osteoporosis and who were at risk of fracture were randomized to a 15-minute infusion of zoledronic acid at a dose of 5 mg (n = 3889) or placebo (n = 3876), given at 12 and 24 months. Over the 3-year study period, treatment with the bisphosphonate resulted in a 70% reduction in the risk of vertebral fracture and a 41% reduction in the risk of hip fracture as compared with placebo (Figure 7.10). The incidences of non-vertebral, clinical and clinical vertebral fractures were also significantly reduced with zoledronic acid treatment compared with placebo, by 25, 33 and 77%, respectively (all $p < 0.001$).

Other key data confirming the efficacy of zoledronic acid in the prevention of fracture come from the HORIZON Recurrent Fracture Study (RFS) [21]. In this study, just over 2000 men and women aged 50 years or older who had been treated for a low-trauma hip fracture were randomized to receive zoledronic acid or placebo a mean of 90 days after surgery. The mean age of the patients was 74.5 years and after a median follow-up of 1.9 years, the rate of any fracture was 8.6% in the zoledronic acid-treated group and 13.9% in the placebo-treated patients (Figure 7.11). This study also reported that significantly fewer patients treated with

Percentage risk of osteoporotic fracture in postmenopausal women treated with zoledronic acid				
	Zoledronic acid	Placebo	RR	95% CI
Incidence of vertebral fracture	3.3	10.9	0.30	0.24–0.38
Incidence of hip fracture	1.4	2.5	0.59	0.42–0.83

Figure 7.10 Percentage risk of osteoporotic fracture in postmenopausal women treated with zoledronic acid. CI, confidence interval; RR, relative risk. Data from the Health Outcomes and Reduced Incidence with Zoledronic Acid Once Yearly (HORIZON) Pivotal Fracture Trial [20].

Effect of zoledronic acid on incidence (%) of fracture in men and women					
	Zoledronic acid	Placebo	RR	95% CI	*p*
Incidence of any fracture (%)	8.6	13.9	0.65	0.50–0.84	0.001
Incidence of nonvertebral fracture (%)	7.6	10.7	0.73	0.55–0.98	0.03
Incidence of hip fracture (%)	2.0	3.5	0.70	0.41–1.19	0.18
Incidence of vertebral fracture (%)	1.7	3.8	0.54	0.32–0.92	0.02

Figure 7.11 Effect of zoledronic acid on incidence (%) of fracture in men and women. CI, confidence interval; RR, relative risk. Data from the Health Outcomes and Reduced Incidence with Zoledronic Acid Once Yearly (HORIZON) Recurrent Fracture Study [21].

the bisphosphonate than with placebo died over the course of the 2-year study, with mortality rates of 9.6% and 13.3%, respectively ($p < 0.01$).

Further support for the use of zoledronic acid was provided by McClung and colleagues [22], who reported that once-yearly zoledronic acid is of benefit in postmenopausal women previously treated with alendronate. In this study, a switch to a single infusion of 5 mg zoledronic acid from the oral bisphosphonate significantly improved BMD at 12 months. Recently, in a 12-month comparator trial in the prevention and treatment of glucocorticoid-induced osteoporosis, Reid et al. [23] have demonstrated superior improvements in BMD at the lumbar spine and total hip in BMD with a single infusion of 5 mg zoledronic acid than with 5 mg or oral daily risedronate. Fractures were very uncommon in the study and there was no significant difference between the two treatment groups.

While zoledronic acid was generally well tolerated in the HORIZON–PFT trial, 1.3% of patients developed atrial fibrillation [20]. This potentially serious adverse effect occurred in 0.5% of placebo-treated patients. The majority of atrial fibrillation cases were observed more than 30 days after the infusion of the bisphosphonate or placebo. Further safety data are therefore awaited and should help more fully assess the long-term clinical safety of this approach [24].

Meta-analyses of bisphosphonates

Among the various pharmacological options, the bisphosphonates appear to provide the greatest antiresorptive efficacy and have become the mainstay in the treatment of postmenopausal osteoporosis [25]. As a class, bisphosphonates significantly suppress bone turnover and increase BMD at the lumbar spine and other sites through their direct inhibitory effect on osteoclasts. Alendronate and risedronate reduce the incidence of vertebral and non-vertebral fractures. Etidronate and ibandronate (oral and intravenous) reduce the incidence of vertebral fractures but their impact on non-vertebral fractures is less clear [26].

The meta-analyses of bisphosphonates are summarized in Figure 7.12 and the common dosing regimens for treatment and prevention of osteoporosis are listed in Figure 7.13.

Tolerability and safety of bisphosphonates

Bisphosphonates are generally well-tolerated and rarely cause toxicity when administered appropriately. In RCTs of oral bisphosphonates, side effects have occurred at similar rates in the active drug and placebo arms [27]. In the 'real-world' setting, however, side effects are relatively common and are a major cause of poor compliance and discontinuation [28].

Meta-analyses of bisphosphonates in the treatment of postmenopausal osteoporosis

Medication	Meta-analyses author	Studies included (n)	Dose	Subjects (n)	Fracture risk reduction (95% CI)		
					Vertebral	Non-vertebral	Hip
Alendronate	Cranney et al. [5]	11	5–40 mg daily	12,855	0.52 (0.43–0.65)	0.51 (0.38–0.69)	NA
Alendronate	Papapoulos et al. [6]	6	5–20 mg daily	9023	NA	NA	0.55 (0.36–0.84)
Risedronate	Cranney et al. [63]	8	2.5–5 mg daily	12,958	0.64 (0.54–0.77)	0.73 (0.61–0.87)	NA
Etidronate	Cranney et al. [10]	13	400 mg daily for 14 days every 3 months	1076	0.63 (0.44–0.92)	0.99 (0.69–1.42)	NA

Figure 7.12 Meta-analyses of bisphosphonates in the treatment of postmenopausal osteoporosis. CI, Confidence interval; NA, not available. Reproduced with permission from Chaiamnuay S, Saag KG. Postmenopausal osteoporosis. What have we learned since the introduction of bisphosphonates? Rev Endocr Metab Disord 2006;7:101–12.

Dosing regimens for commonly utilized bisphosphonates in treatment and prevention of osteoporosis

Bisphosphonate	Treatment dose	Prevention dose
Alendronate	70 mg oral weekly	35 oral weekly *
	10 mg oral daily	5 mg oral daily
Risedronate	35 mg oral weekly	35 mg oral weekly
	5 mg oral daily	5 mg oral daily
Ibrandronate	150 mg oral monthly	150 mg oral monthly
	3 mg intravenous (over 15–30 s) every 3 months **	
Etidronate	400 mg oral once daily for 14 days every 3 months	Same as treatment dose

Figure 7.13 Dosing regimens for commonly utilized bisphosphonates in treatment and prevention of osteoporosis. * In US market. ** Available in Canada and Europe. Reproduced with permission from Chaiamnuay S, Saag KG. Postmenopausal osteoporosis. What have we learned since the introduction of bisphosphonates? Rev Endocr Metab Disord 2006;7:101–12.

Gastrointestinal side effects

The most frequent side effects of oral bisphosphonates involve the upper GI tract and include nausea, diarrhoea, gastritis and oesphageal irritation. Gastric and duodenal ulcers have also been reported [29]. The mechanism appears to be related to direct irritation and erosive action on the mucosa; for instance, alendronate crystalline material has been found in the biopsies of patients with alendronate-induced oesophagitis and gastric ulcer [26]. Upper GI symptoms tend to be more common in patients with a history of upper GI disorders and those taking concomitant non-steroidal anti-inflammatory agents, proton pump inhibitors or histamine-receptor blockers.

Because oral bisphosphonates interact with food and drink, they are subject to strict dosing requirements. They must be taken on an empty stomach, at least half an hour before eating, and the patient must remain upright for at least 30 minutes after dosing. Contraindications to oral bisphosphonates therapy include abnormalities of the oesophagus that delay emptying (e.g. stricture, dysmotility or achalasia), low serum calcium, severe renal dysfunction (creatinine clearance <35 mL/min), and an inability to maintain an upright posture (sitting or standing) for at least 30 minutes after oral administration. Consequently, oral bisphosphonates cannot be used in bed-bound patients, despite this group being at high risk for osteoporosis. Bisphosphonates are also contraindicated in women who are pregnant or nursing.

There are various explanations for the discrepancy between the incidence of upper GI side effects in the community compared with clinical trials. Some RCTs excluded patients with upper GI risk factors or a history of peptic ulcers. Other possibilities for the increased rate of GI side effects in the community are poor adherence to the manufacturer's instructions on proper bisphosphonate administration, a higher background prevalence of GI tract disorders among older women, and increased awareness of GI side effects leading to increased reporting of events [25,30].

The GI side effects associated with oral bisphosphonates have led to interest in alternative administration regimens, including intermittent and intravenous dosing. These options are discussed in Chapter 8.

Osteonecrosis of the jaw

Since 2004, cases of osteonecrosis of the jaw have been increasingly reported in patients treated with bisphosphonates; most of these patients were receiving the bisphosphonate for bone metastasis or myeloma, but for a small number it was for osteoporosis. Based on current evidence the risk in osteoporosis appears to be comparable to that in the general population. It is likely that osteonecrosis of the jaw results from direct toxicity to cells of bone and soft tissue from high-potency bisphosphonates, probably acting through their effects on the mevalonate pathway [31]. A typical presentation is a non-healing tooth-extraction socket or exposed jawbone, which is refractory to conservative debridement and antibiotic therapy.

Oversuppression of bone turnover

Bisphosphonates are potent inhibitors of bone resorption and have a very long skeletal half-life, raising concerns that their long-term use might impair bone strength. Evidence from animal models suggests that bisphosphonates might inhibit the normal repair of bone microdamage. In addition, oversuppression of bone turnover may produce hypermineralized, brittle bone [26].

Etidronate is known to cause abnormal mineralization of bone, resembling osteomalacia, when given continuously for long periods. To reduce this risk etidronate is administered as intermittent, low cyclical doses, a regimen that is supported by long-term safety data [9]. On the other hand, a study of alendronate given continuously for 10 years indicated that treatment was safe and offered sustained benefits in terms of BMD and remodelling, with no decrease in antifracture efficacy [32]. However there have been recent reports of an increased incidence of subtrochanteric or proximal diaphyseal femur fractures [33,34]. Although these reports are of concern, an increased prevalence in a population register has not been confirmed [35].

Other side effects

Bisphosphonates have also been associated with adverse central nervous system effects, such as hallucinations (auditory and olfactory) and ocular disturbances (conjunctivitis, blurred vision, eye pain and inflammation). Although rare, these side effects can lead to serious problems. Recent reports of atrial fibrillation (AF) occurring as serious adverse event in the zoledronic acid HORIZON Pivotal Fracture Trial [20] were not confirmed in the HORIZON Recurrent Fracture Study [21]. Furthermore, a recently reported prescription database study from Denmark, while suggesting that AF was-more common in bisphosphonates users, suggested that this was more likely due to comorbidity in those prescribed bisphosphonates rather than the drugs themselves [36].

Oestrogen

Oestrogen deficiency is a leading cause of osteoporosis and the positive effect of oestrogen replacement therapy on BMD is well-established (Figure 7.14). More than 50 RCTs have shown that oestrogen, either unopposed or combined with a progesterone derivative, is effective in increasing spine and hip BMD. Furthermore, oestrogen replacement therapy has been shown to reduce the risk of non-vertebral and hip fracture in women with postmenopausal osteoporosis [37,38].

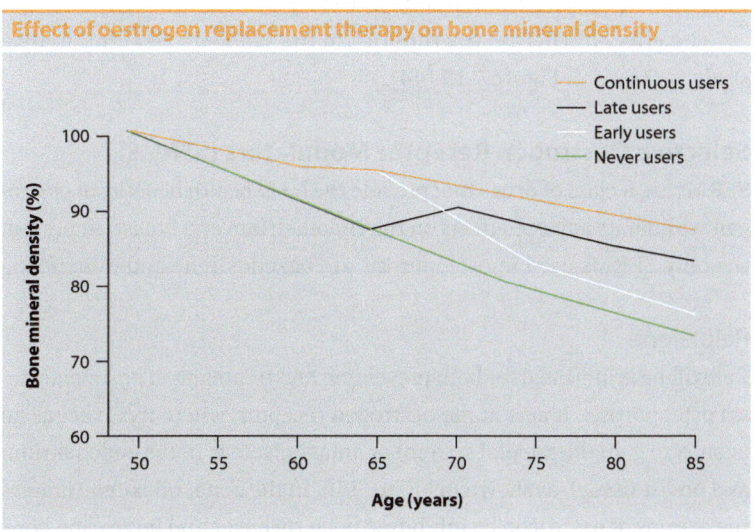

Effect of oestrogen replacement therapy on bone mineral density

Figure 7.14 **Effect of oestrogen replacement therapy on bone mineral density**. Adapted with permission from Levine JP. Long-term estrogen and hormone replacement therapy for the prevention and treatment of osteoporosis. Curr Womens Health Rep 2003; 3:181–6.

Until December 2003, oestrogen-containing hormone replacement therapy (HRT) was considered the first-line treatment for preventing osteoporosis in postmenopausal women. However, this changed following the publication of two large randomized controlled studies. Both the Women's Health Initiative study [39] and the Million Women Study [40] found that women taking combined oestrogen/progestin HRT had a significantly increased risk of breast cancer compared with those taking placebo. In addition, HRT is associated with an increased risk of endometrial cancer and venous thromboembolism (VTE) and, contrary to previous reports, does not appear to protect against heart disease or cognitive decline [41,42].

In the light of this new evidence as well as the introduction of several new effective therapies for osteoporosis, HRT ceased to be a first-line therapy for the prevention of osteoporosis in women aged over 50 years [43]. However it remains an option for women intolerant of, or refractory to, other therapies, and for the prevention of osteoporosis in women with premature menopause and aged 50 years or less. In addition, HRT is still recommended for the treatment of menopausal symptoms that adversely affect quality of life; treatment should be given at the minimum effective dose and for the shortest duration of time [43].

The effect of HRT on fracture risk in the Women's Health Initiative study is shown in Figure 7.15 [44].

Selective Oestrogen Receptor Modulators (SERMs)

SERMs are a class of drugs that provide the bone health benefits of oestrogen without its adverse effects on the endometrium and breast. At present the only SERMs used in osteoporosis are bazedoxifene and raloxifene.

Raloxifene

Raloxifene is indicated for both prevention and treatment of postmenopausal osteoporosis. It acts at the oestrogen receptor, where it can act as an agonist (e.g. in the skeletal system) or antagonist (e.g. in the endometrium and breast tissue), as shown in Figure 7.16. In the bone, raloxifene mimics the actions of oestrogen by inhibiting bone turnover and increasing bone density. Secondary benefits of raloxifene include its cholesterol-lowering properties and a potential reduction in the risk of breast cancer.

Cumulative risk of fracture in the Women's Health Initiative study: Kaplan–Meier estimates of hazard

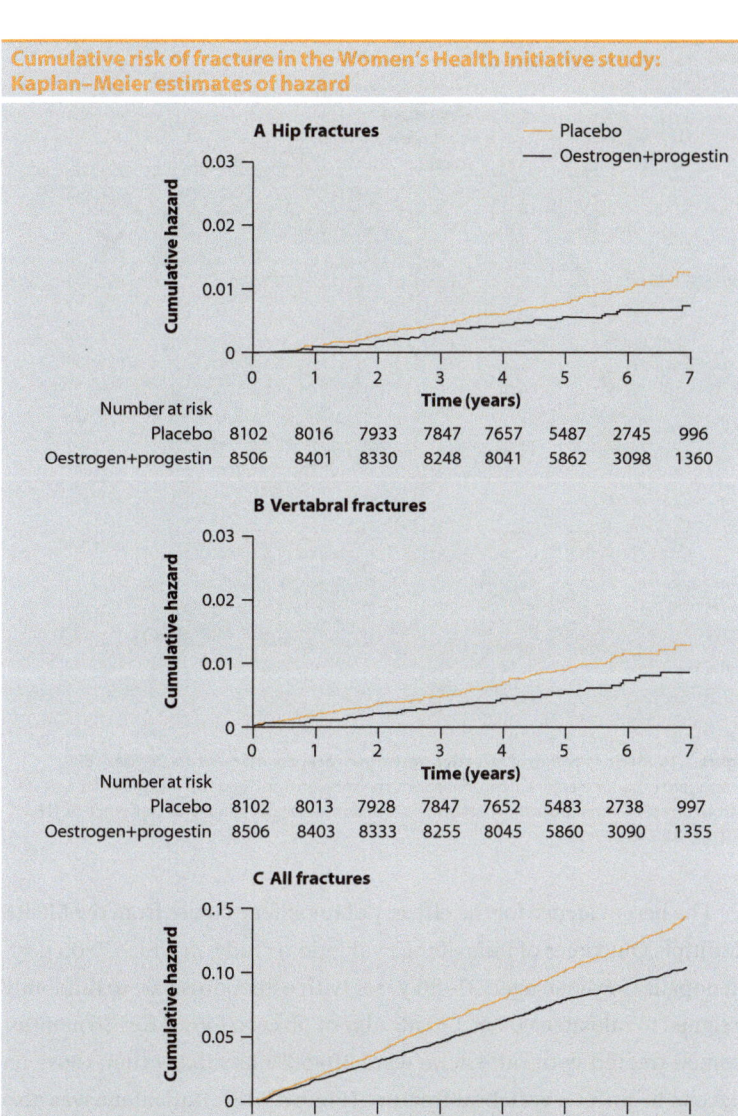

Figure 7.15 Cumulative risk of fracture in the Women's Health Initiative study: Kaplan–Meier estimates of hazard. Reproduced with permission from Cauley JA, Robbins J, Chen Z, et al. Effects of estrogen plus progestin on risk of fracture and bone mineral density. The Women's Health Initiative Randomized Trial. JAMA 2003; 290:1729–38.

Mode of action of selective oestrogen receptor modulators (SERMs)

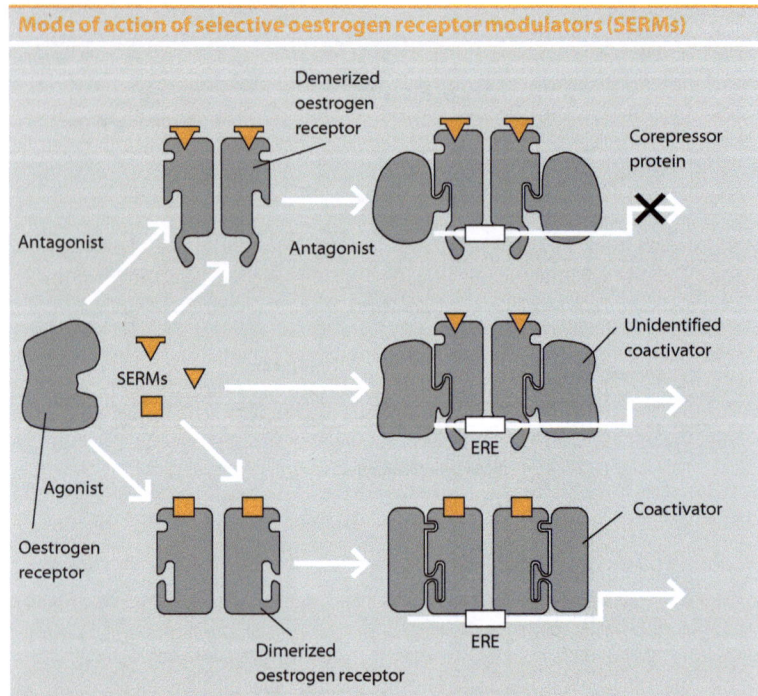

Figure 7.16 Mode of action of selective oestrogen receptor modulators (SERMs). ERE, Oestrogen response element. Reproduced with permission from Riggs BL, Hartmann LC. Selective estrogen-receptor modulators – mechanisms of action and application to clinical practice. N Engl J Med 2003; 348:618–29.

The best evidence for the efficacy of raloxifene comes from the MORE (Multiple Outcomes of Raloxifene Evaluation) study, in which 7705 postmenopausal women aged 31–80 years with osteoporosis were randomly assigned to raloxifene 60 or 120 mg/day or placebo [45]. After 36 months, women treated with raloxifene were 30–50% less likely than those on placebo to suffer a vertebral fracture (Figure 7.17). Raloxifene was also associated with significant increases in BMD at the hip and spine, and with reductions in blood and urine markers of bone turnover [46].

Eight-year follow-up of participants in the MORE study identified no increased risk of myocardial infarction, stroke, uterine cancer, endometrial hyperplasia, ovarian cancer, breast tenderness or postmenopausal bleeding associated with raloxifene therapy [47].

The cardiovascular safety of raloxifene was also investigated in the RUTH (Raloxifene Use for the Heart) study [48]. In this RCT, more than 10,000 postmenopausal women with established coronary heart disease (CHD) or multiple CHD risk factors were randomized to raloxifene 60 mg/day or placebo and followed for a median of 5.9 years. Raloxifene had no effect on the risk of CHD events but significantly reduced the risk of invasive breast cancer and vertebral fracture. However, raloxifene was associated with an increased risk of fatal stroke and venous thromboembolism (VTE).

The most common adverse effects of raloxifene are hot flushes and muscle cramps. Raloxifene is contraindicated in patients with a history of VTE and during periods of prolonged immobilization.

Bazedoxifene

Another SERM, bazedoxifene, has been approved for use in Europe and is currently under review by the US Food and Drug Administration. Bazedoxifene has a similar mechanism of action to raloxifene and also has been shown to reduce low-density lipoprotein (LDL) and total cholesterol and raise high-density lipoprotein (HDL) cholesterol [49].

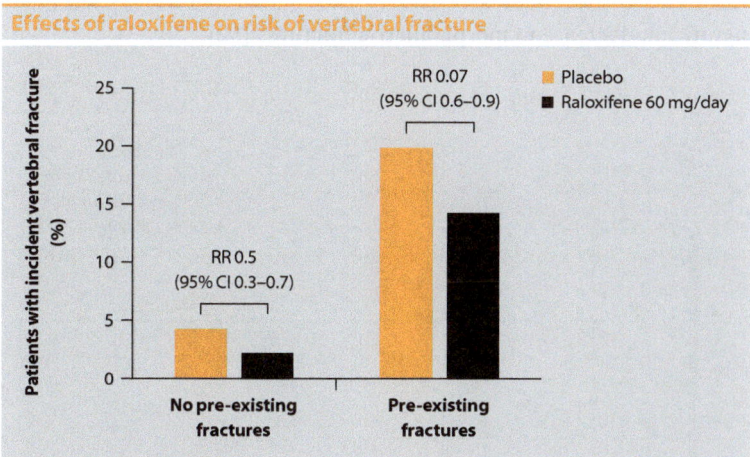

Figure 7.17 Effects of raloxifene on risk of vertebral fracture. Reproduced with permission from Ettinger B, Black DM, Mitlak BH, et al. Reduction of vertebral fracture risk in postmenopausal women with osteoporosis treated with raloxifene: results from a 3-year randomized clinical trial. JAMA 1999; 282:637–45.

In a 2-year, multicentre, placebo-controlled trial, 1583 postmenopausal women aged ≥45 years at risk for osteoporosis were randomized to receive bazedoxifene 10, 20 or 40 mg/day, raloxifene 60 mg/day or placebo. At the end of the study period, lumbar spine BMD was significantly greater in all three bazedoxifene groups than in the placebo group ($p < 0.001$) and was comparable to raloxifene (Figure 7.18). Similar results were seen for total hip BMD. Patients taking bazedoxifene or raloxifene also had significant reductions in serum bone markers compared with those taking placebo ($p < 0.001$). Bazedoxifene was generally safe and well tolerated; the most common adverse events were hot flushes and leg cramps [50].

Bazedoxifene has also been shown to reduce new vertebral fracture risk in patients who already have osteoporosis. In a 3-year study of nearly 7500 women randomized to receive bazedoxifene 20 or 40 mg/day, raloxifene 60 mg/day, or placebo, the incidence of new vertebral fracture was significantly lower in the raloxifene and both bazedoxifene groups than in the placebo group ($p < 0.05$) (Figure 7.19). There were no significant differences between the bazedoxifene and raloxifene groups [51]. A post hoc analysis of this study found that in just the patients taking bazedoxifene, there was a non-significant trend towards a decrease in clinical fractures (hazard ratio 0.84; 95% CI 0.67–1.06, $p = 0.14$) and a significant decrease in morphometric fractures [52].

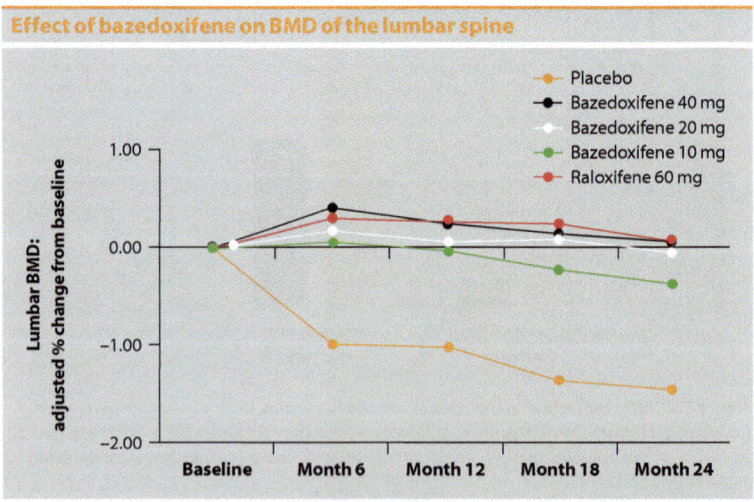

Figure 7.18 Effect of bazedoxifene on BMD of the lumbar spine. Data from Miller et al. [50].

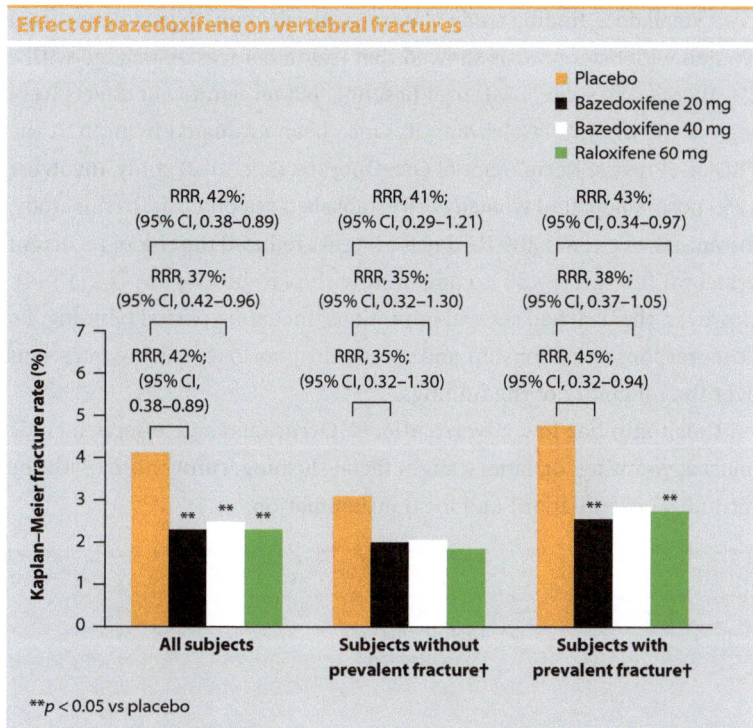

Figure 7.19 Effect of bazedoxifene on vertebral fractures. Incidence of new fractures is given in relation to baseline fracture status. The intent-to-treat population was 6847 patients. †$p = 0.89$ for treatment by prevalent fracture status intervention. CI, confidence interval; RRR, relative risk reduction. Data from Silverman et al. [51].

Calcitonin

Calcitonin is an endogenous hormone that helps regulate calcium levels through a negative feedback mechanism. It lowers circulating calcium levels by suppressing osteoclast activity, thereby inhibiting bone loss. It also reduces tubular reabsorption of calcium in the kidneys (Figure 7.20).

Calcitonin is approved for treatment but not prevention of postmenopausal osteoporosis. It is less effective than other pharmacologic therapies for osteoporosis and is thus reserved for second- or third-line use. It is recommended for use in women with osteoporosis who are at least 5 years past menopause. Most calcitonin products consist of salmon calcitonin, either obtained directly from salmon or chemically synthesized.

A small dose-finding study of intranasal calcitonin in postmenopausal women with osteoporosis showed that treatment was associated with a 3% increase in spinal BMD over baseline; but no significant effects were seen at the hip [53]. Calcitonin has also been evaluated in an RCT, the PROOF (Prevent Recurrence of OsteOporotic Fractures) study, involving 1255 postmenopausal women with established osteoporosis. In this study, intranasal calcitonin 200 IU/day for 5 years reduced the risk of recurrent vertebral fracture by 33% compared with placebo (Figure 7.21) [54]. However, the trial had several limitations, including partial blinding, no dose–response relationship and a 60% dropout rate, raising questions over the reliability of the findings.

Calcitonin has few adverse effects. Occasional side effects include nausea, vomiting, dizziness, slight facial flushing, runny nose (with the intranasal formulation) and local inflammation.

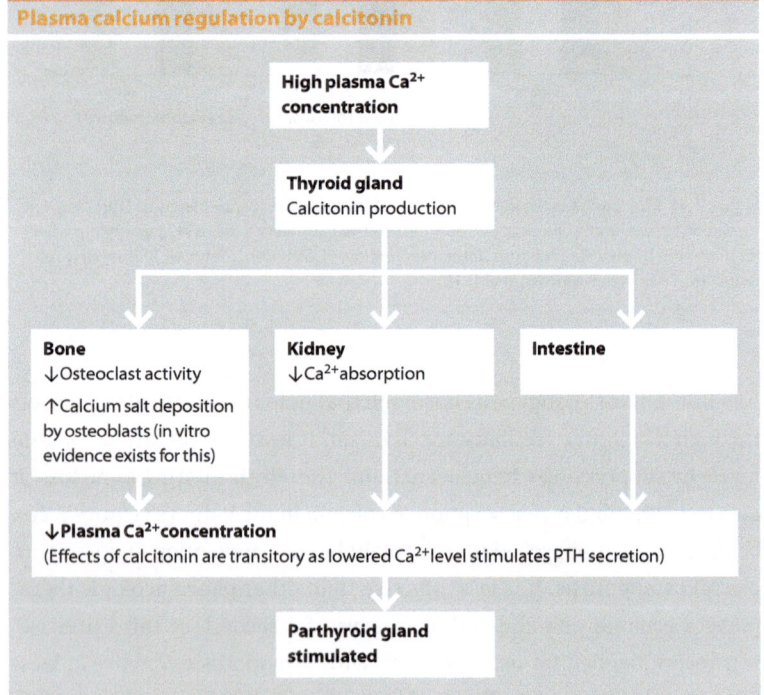

Figure 7.20 Plasma calcium regulation by calcitonin. PTH, parathyroid hormone.

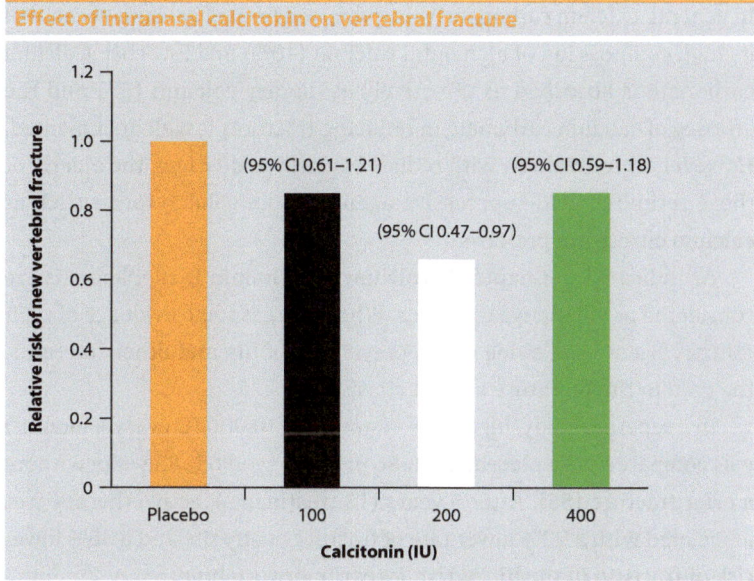

Figure 7.21 Effect of intranasal calcitonin on vertebral fracture. CI, Confidence interval. Reproduced with permission from Chesnut CH III, Silverman S, Andriano K, et al. A randomized trial of nasal spray salmon calcitonin in postmenopausal women with established osteoporosis: the Prevent Recurrence of Osteoporotic Fractures Study. PROOF study group. Am J Med 2000;109:267–76.

Calcium plus vitamin D

All women receiving pharmacological treatment for osteoporosis should be calcium- and vitamin D-replete. The recommended dietary intake in postmenopausal women is calcium ≥ 1200 mg/day and vitamin D_3 400–800 IU/day. Supplementation is accepted adjunctive treatment for osteoporosis and may also be used as a preventive measure. Daily calcium and vitamin D_3 supplementation is also recommended for elderly institutionalized people with limited exposure to sunlight.

More than 100 different formulations of calcium and vitamin D_3 are available worldwide. Their efficacy is related to dosage, mode of administration and the type of calcium salt used in the preparation. For instance, a single tablet containing both calcium and vitamin D_3 is better tolerated than separate formulations [55], and chewable calcium tablets are more acceptable to patients than soluble or effervescent forms [56].

In general, calcium carbonate is the preferred form of calcium because of its high composition of elemental calcium (40%) and low cost. Calcium carbonate is absorbed as effectively as dietary calcium [57] and the efficacy of calcium carbonate in reducing fractures is well documented. However, in individuals with reduced gastric acidity (e.g. the elderly or those receiving acid-suppressive agents), more soluble forms such as calcium citrate are preferred.

As indicated in Chapter 6, calcium and vitamin D supplements are considered as adjunctive therapies. While there is some evidence of their efficacy when used alone in the prevention of hip and other fractures, the data in the literature are not consistent.

In a separate study, high-dose vitamin D_3 (10,000 IU every 4 months) was compared with placebo in 2686 patients aged 65–85 years without a prior fracture [58]. After 5 years (15 treatments), active therapy was associated with a 22% lower rate of fracture at any site and a 33% lower risk of fracture in the hip, wrist, forearm, or vertebrae.

Calcium and vitamin D_3 supplements are generally well tolerated. Excessive intake of calcium (>2000 mg/day for most patients) may cause constipation, dyspepsia and hypercalciuria. Excessive vitamin D_3 intake (>2000 IU/day for most patients) should be avoided as it may lead to hypercalcaemia, hypercalciuria, polyuria, renal stones, renal failure and ectopic calcium deposition.

Parathyroid hormone derivatives

Parathyroid hormone (PTH) is a major endogenous regulator of calcium and phosphate homeostasis. The body's response to PTH is complex but in general terms is aimed at increasing calcium levels in the extracellular fluid. PTH acts at three main sites in the body: the bone, kidney and intestines (Figure 7.22).

Teriparatide is a synthetic version of the first 34 amino acids from the *N*-terminal portion of PTH. It has been shown to stimulate bone formation, thereby increasing bone mass and strength as well as improving calcium balance [59]. It is approved for the treatment of severe/established osteoporosis in postmenopausal women. Teriparatide is administered parenterally and treatment duration was initially restricted to

18 months in Europe but this has now been extended to 24 months in line with the US licence.

In a RCT involving 1637 postmenopausal women with a previous vertebral fracture, 19 months of treatment with subcutaneous teriparatide 20 or 40 μg/day reduced the incidence of vertebral fractures by 65 and 69%, respectively, and non-vertebral fractures by 53 and 54%, respectively, compared with placebo (Figures 7.23 and 7.24) [60]. Active therapy also increased BMD in the spine, hip and radius significantly more than placebo.

Teriparatide appears to have less effect on cortical than trabecular bone [61], suggesting that its main use will be in preventing vertebral rather than hip fractures.

Teriparatide is generally well tolerated. The most common adverse reactions are gastrointestinal (GI) disturbances, pain at the injection site, headache and orthostatic hypotension. Teriparatide is contraindicated in

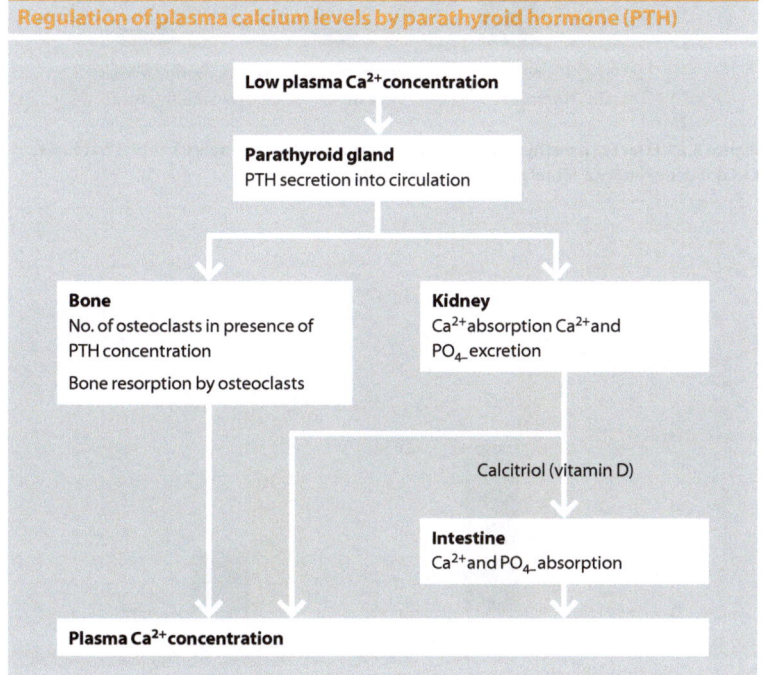

Figure 7.22 Regulation of plasma calcium levels by parathyroid hormone (PTH).

patients at increased risk of osteosarcoma, having been shown to cause osteosarcoma in growing male and female rats. There has been no evidence in trials or clinical practice as yet of osteosarcoma developing in humans related to the therapy. Teriperatide is also contraindicated in those with metabolic bone disease including Paget's disease and hyperparathyroidism.

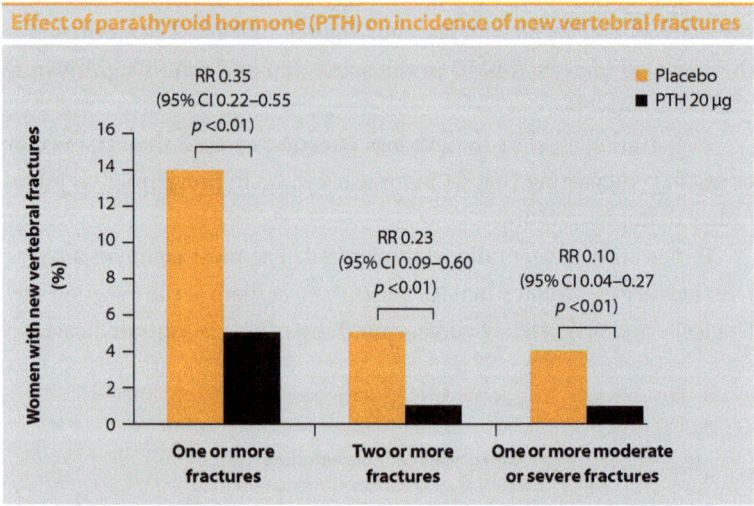

Figure 7.23 Effect of parathyroid hormone (PTH) on incidence of new vertebral fractures. CI, Confidence interval; RR, relative risk. Data from Neer et al. [60].

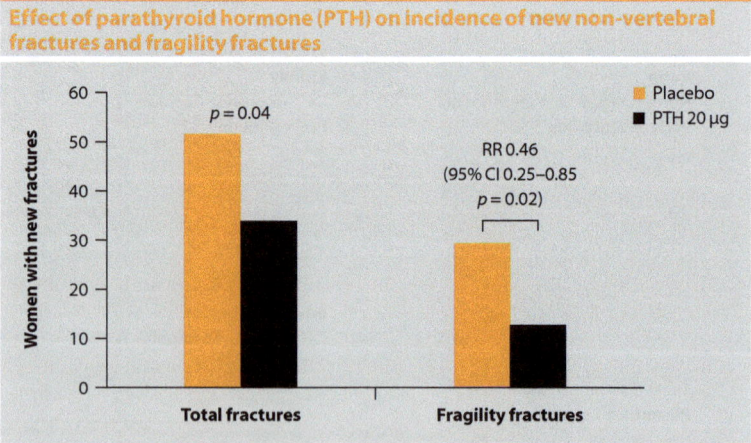

Figure 7.24 Effect of parathyroid hormone (PTH) on incidence of new non-vertebral fractures and fragility fractures. CI, Confidence interval; RR, relative risk. Data from Neer et al. [60].

Data have also been published demonstrating the value of full-length synthetic PTH (1-84). 2532 postmenopausal women with BMD at the hip or lumbar spine received 100 μg of recombinant human PTH or placebo daily by subcutaneous injection plus calcium and vitamin D_3 400 U/day. Parathyroid hormone reduced the risk for new or worsened vertebral fractures by 58% (relative risk 0.42; 95% CI, 0.24–0.72; $p = 0.001$). However only 67% of subjects completed the 18-month trial and when the relative risk reduction was recalculated for those who completed the trial it was 0.60 (95%CI 0.36–1.00; $p = 0.050$) [46]. While there were significant increases in BMD at the spine and at the hip, parathyroid hormone treatment increased the percentage of participants with hypercalcaluria, hypercalcaemia, and nausea [62]. Nevertheless the 1–84 version of recombinant PTH is available in some countries for use over an 18-month period.

Strontium ranelate

Strontium ranelate is the first in a new class of drugs which, although primarily antiresoptive, has some anabolic properties [63]. It causes bone turnover to be rebalanced in favour of bone formation, resulting in increased bone strength (Figure 7.25) [64,65].

The efficacy of strontium ranelate in reducing fractures at the spine and hip has been demonstrated in several large phase III clinical trials. In the SOTI (Spinal Osteoporosis Therapeutic Intervention) study, 1649 postmenopausal women with osteoporosis and at least one vertebral fracture were randomized to strontium ranelate 2 g/day or placebo for 3 years [66]. Active therapy was associated with a 49% risk reduction for new vertebral fractures, as well as increases in BMD of 14.4% at the spine and 8.3% at the hip. The benefits were apparent after just 1 year and were sustained for the study duration (Figure 7.26).

PREVOS (PREVention Of early postmenopausal bone loss by Strontium ranelate) was a placebo-controlled dose-ranging study conducted in 160 early postmenopausal women without osteoporosis [67]. After 2 years, lumbar BMD increased by 5.3% over baseline values among women receiving strontium ranelate 1 g/day, but it was unchanged in placebo-treated women.

The increases in BMD in this study and all others using strontium ranelate are larger than expected, due in part to the greater attenuation of strontium than calcium hence giving artificially higher BMD values [68].

More recently, the TROPOS (TReatment Of Peripheral. OSteoporosis) study involved 5091 postmenopausal women with osteoporosis aged 75 years and over [69]. Compared with placebo, 3 years of treatment with strontium ranelate 2 g/day was associated with a 16% reduction in non-vertebral fractures, 19% reduction in major fragility fractures, 36% reduction in hip fractures, 39% reduction in vertebral fractures, and an increase in BMD of 8.2% at the femoral neck and 9.8% at the total hip (Figure 7.27).

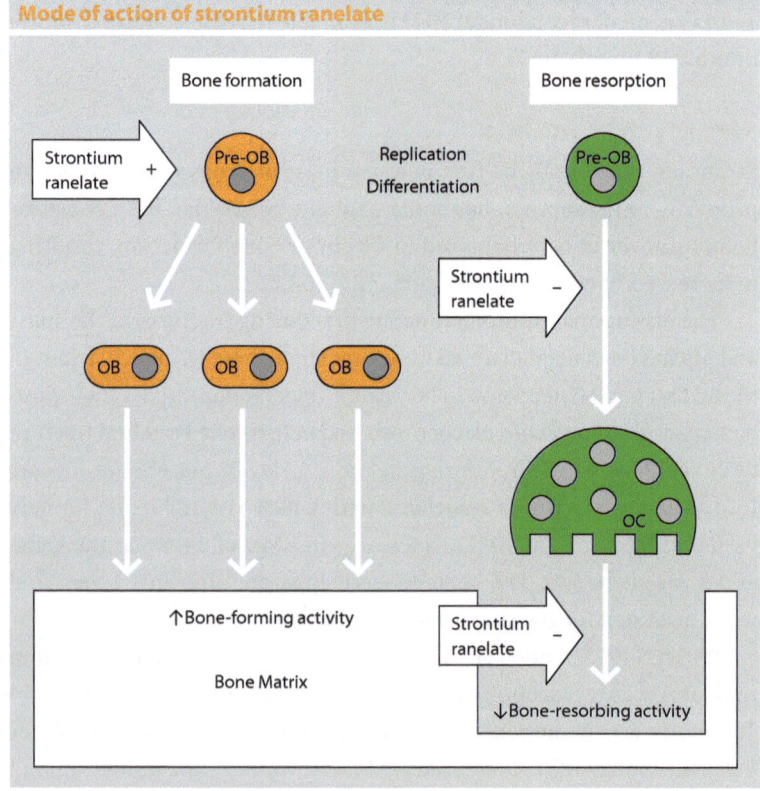

Figure 7.25 Mode of action of strontium ranelate. OC, Osteoclast; OB, osteoblast. Reproduced with permission from Marie PJ, Ammann P, Boivin G, et al. Mechanisms of action and therapeutical potential of strontium in bone. Calcif Tissue Int 2001; 69:121–9.

In these clinical trials strontium ranelate was generally well tolerated, with an incidence of side effects comparable to placebo. The most common side effects were nausea and diarrhoea; as with other side effects these tended to be mild and transient. Due to a small increase in the risk of VTE, strontium ranelate should be used with caution in patients at risk of this condition.

The recommended dose for strontium ranelate is one 2g sachet daily, by mouth. Because absorption of strontium ranelate is slow and is reduced by food, it should be taken at least 2 hours after eating, preferably at night.

Denosumab

Denosumab is a fully human monoclonal immunoglobulin G2 (IgG2) antibody directed against RANKL [70]. This novel agent is currently under investigation for the treatment and prevention of postmenopausal osteoporosis [71,72], rheumatoid arthritis [73], treatment-induced bone loss, bone metastases and multiple myeloma [70].

A recent phase III trial, Fracture Reduction Evaluation of Denosumab in Osteoporosis Every 6 months (FREEDOM), reported a significant reduction in the risk of vertebral, non-vertebral and hip fracture with denosumab

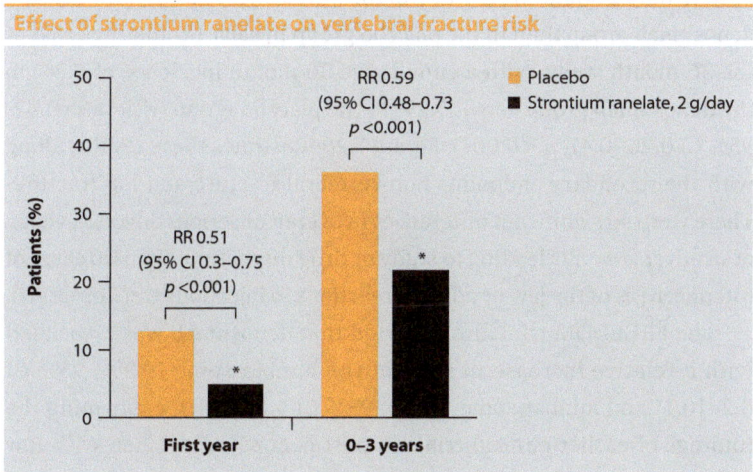

Figure 7.26 Effect of strontium ranelate on vertebral fracture risk. CI, Confidence interval; RR, relative risk. Adapted with permission from Meunier PJ, Roux C, Seeman E, et al. The effects of strontium ranelate on the risk of vertebral fracture in women with postmenopausal osteoporosis. N Engl J Med 2004; 350:459–68.

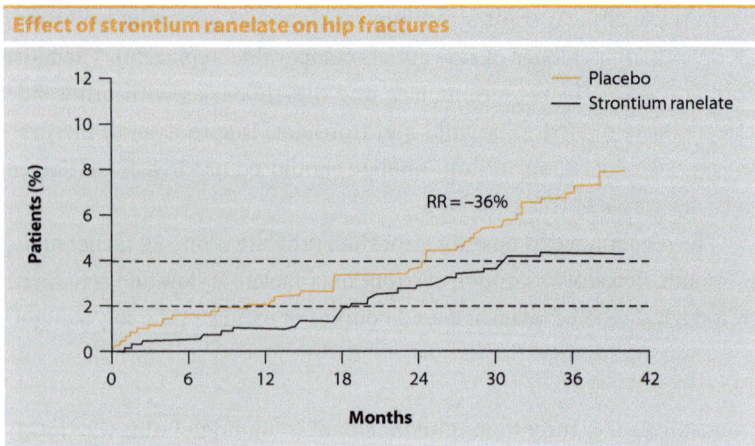

Figure 7.27 Effect of strontium ranelate on hip fractures. Reproduced with permission from Rizzoli R. Atlas of Postmenopausal Osteoporosis, 2nd edition. London: Current Medicine Group Limited, 2005.

[74]. Eligible patients were aged 60– 90 years and had T-score of less than –2.5 and more than –4.0 at the lumbar spine or hip. In total, 7868 patients were randomized to receive 60 mg of denosumab or placebo subcutaneously every 6 months for 36 months. The primary endpoint, incidence of new radiographic vertebral fracture, was significantly lower in the denosumab group than in the placebo group in each 12-month period of the 36-month study, with a cumulative 36-month incidence of 2.3% in the denosumab group versus 7.2% in the placebo group (risk ratio 0.32, 95% CI 0.26–0.41, p <0.001). Figure 7.28 illustrates these results, along with the secondary endpoints non-vertebral fracture and hip fracture. There were no significant differences in overall or serious adverse events, or in adverse events leading to study or drug discontinuation. No cases of osteonecrosis of the jaw or adverse reactions to injections were observed.

The FREEDOM trial also reported that denosumab was associated with a relative increase in BMD at the lumbar spine (9.2%; 95% CI 8.2–10.1) and lumbar spine (6.0%; 95% CI 5.2–6.7%), confirming the findings of earlier clinical trials in postmenopausal women with low BMD. For example, in one trial subcutaneous injection of denosumab every 3–6 months for up to 2 years was found to significantly increase BMD at the lumbar spine, total hip, distal one-third radius, and total

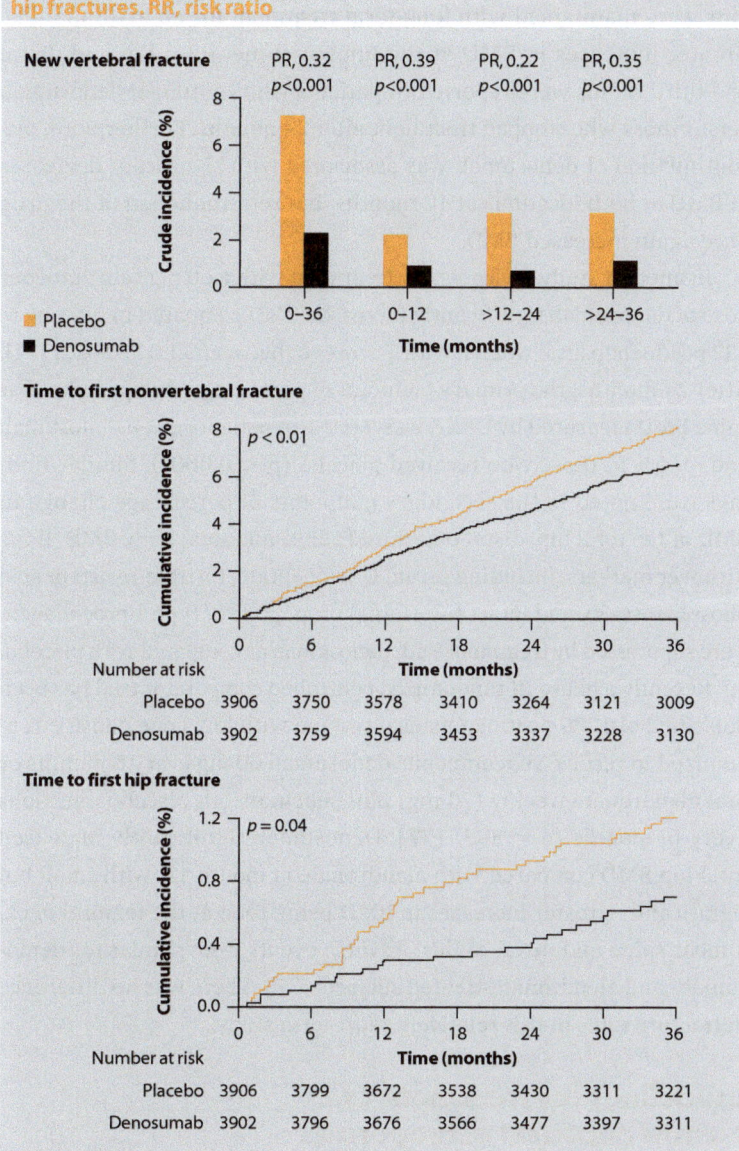

Figure 7.28 Effect of denosumab on incidence of new vertebral, non-vertebral and hip fractures. RR, risk ratio. Reproduced with permission from Cummings SR, San Martin J, McClung MR, et al. Denosumab for prevention of fractures in postmenopausal women with osteoporosis. N Engl J Med 2009;361:756–65.

body [75,76]. An extended phase II study [72] showed that these benefits were maintained with long-term treatment for up to 48 months. Greater increases in BMD at the lumbar spine, total hip and distal one-third radius were reported in patients who continued denosumab versus those who stopped treatment after 24 months. Furthermore, discontinuation of denosumab was associated with significant decreases in BMD at both locations at 12 months, but reintroduction of the drug once again increased BMD.

In another study, twice-yearly treatment with a 60 mg subcutaneous dose of denosumab significantly increased BMD compared to placebo in 332 postmenopausal women with T-scores of between –1.0 and –2.5 [71]. After 24 months, the primary endpoint of percentage change in lumbar spine BMD measured by DEXA was +6.0% in patients given denosumab and –0.6% in those who received placebo ($p < 0.0001$). Similar findings were noted in the secondary endpoints of percentage change in BMD at the total hip, distal one-third radius, and total body BMD. Bone turnover markers, including serum C-telopeptide, tartrate-resistant acid phosphatase-5b, and intact N-terminal propeptide of type 1 procollagen, were suppressed by treatment with denosumab as compared with placebo.

Recently a phase III randomized controlled comparator trial has been published of 1289 postmenopausal women with low bone density, randomized to receive subcutaneous denosumab 60 mg every 6 months or oral alendronate weekly (70 mg) plus subcutaneous placebo injections every 6 months (n = 595) [77]. Denosumab significantly increased total hip BMD compared with alendronate at month 12, with small but significantly greater increases in BMD being seen at the femoral neck, lumbar spine and distal radius. Adverse events were similar for demosumab- and alendronate-treated subjects [77]. There was no difference in fracture rates in this relatively short-term study.

Guidelines for treatment of postmenopausal osteoporosis

Bisphosphonates are currently the treatment of choice in women based on their efficacy and their very low cost, with alendronate now being available generically [25]. In the United Kingdom, for example, evidence-based guidance or guidelines issued by the National Institute for Health and Clinical Excellence (NICE), the Scottish Intercollegiate Guidelines Network (SIGN) and the National Osteoporosis Guidelines group recommend bisphosphonates as first-line treatment options in postmenopausal women with osteoporosis [2,78]. These guidelines define the circumstances under which women are eligible for treatment and state that the choice of bisphosphonate is at the prescribing physician's discretion, taking into account the individual patient's medical history and preferences as well as the drug's proven effectiveness profile, cost, tolerability and safety. As well as bisphosphonates, these guidelines endorse the use of other pharmacological options under specific circumstances, including raloxifene, strontium ranelate, teriparatide and in some cases HRT and combination therapy. NICE is currently reconsidering its guidance for the use of strontium ranelate as well as the bisphosphonates and teriparatide in the prevention and treatment of postmenopausal osteoporosis [30,79].

Current thinking about combination therapy

Combining therapies in an attempt to achieve greater benefit is common in medical practice. In clinical trials, bisphosphonates, raloxifene and calcitonin have usually been assessed in combination with calcium and/or vitamin D. Therefore patients receiving any of these drugs should be calcium- and vitamin D-replete, by means of supplementation if dietary intake is insufficient.

Bisphosphonates have been studied in combination with other drugs, including oestrogen-containing HRT, raloxifene and PTH. The duration of therapy and order of use (i.e. sequential versus add-on) has varied from study to study. In some cases combination therapy has been associated with significantly greater increases in BMD than has either agent alone. Some combinations have also been found to suppress markers of bone turnover more than monotherapy.

To date however, in terms of fracture rates, combination therapy has not demonstrated a significant benefit in comparison with single agents. Furthermore, it is clear that combination treatment will increase cost, and it is possible that it will increase side effects and reduce therapy adherence. Given the absence of a demonstrable clinical benefit and the potential disadvantages in terms of cost and tolerability, combination therapy is not currently recommended.

References

1 Dawson-Hughes B, Lindsay R, Khosla S, et al. National Osteoporosis Foundation Clinician's Guide to Prevention and Treatment of Osteoporosis. Washington: National Osteoporosis Foundation 2008 Available from http://www.nof.org/Professionals/Clinicians_Guide.htm [last accessed 7th October 2009].

2 Compston J, Cooper A, Cooper C, et al. Guidelines for the diagnosis and management of osteoporosis in postmenopausal women and men from the age of 50 years in the UK. Maturitas 2009;62:105–8.

3 Cummings SR, Black DM, Thompson DE, et al. Effect of alendronate on risk of fracture in women with low bone density but without vertebral fractures: results from the Fracture Intervention Trial. JAMA 1998;280:2077–82.

4 Black DM, Cummings SR, Karpf DB, et al. Randomised trial of effect of alendronate on risk of fracture in women with existing vertebral fractures. Fracture Intervention Trial Research Group. Lancet 1996;348:1535–41.

5 Cranney A, Wells G, Willan A, et al. Meta-analyses of therapies for postmenopausal osteoporosis. II. Meta-analysis of alendronate for the treatment of postmenopausal women. Endocrine Rev 2002;23:508–16.

6 Papapoulos SE, Quandt SA, Liberman UA, et al. Meta-analysis of the efficacy of alendronate for the prevention of hip fractures in postmenopausal women. Osteoporos Int 2005;16:468–74.

7 Schnitzer T, Bone HG, Crepaldi G, et al. Therapeutic equivalence of alendronate 70 mg once-weekly and alendronate 10 mg daily in the treatment of osteoporosis. Alendronate Once-Weekly Study Group. Aging 2000;12:1–12.

8 Watts NB, Harris ST, Genant HK, et al. Intermittent cyclical etidronate treatment of postmenopausal osteoporosis. N Engl J Med 1990;323:73–9.

9 Miller PD, Watts NB, Licata AA, et al. Cyclical etidronate in the treatment of postmenopausal osteoporosis: efficacy and safety after seven years of treatment. Am J Med 1997;103:46–76.

10 Cranney A, Guyatt G, Krolicki N, et al. A meta-analysis of etidronate for the treatment of postmenopausal osteoporosis. Osteoporos Int 2001;12:140–51.

11 Chesnut III CH, Skag A, Christiansen C, et al. Effects of oral ibandronate administered daily or intermittently on fracture risk in postmenopausal osteoporosis. J Bone Miner Res 2004;19:1241–9.

12 Reginster JY, Adami S, Lakatos P, et al. Efficacy and tolerability of once-monthly oral ibandronate in postmenopausal osteoporosis: 2 year results from the MOBILE study. Ann Rheum Dis 2006;65:654–61.

13 Delmas PD, Adami S, Strugala C, et al. Intravenous ibandronate injections in postmenopausal women with osteoporosis: one-year results from the dosing intravenous administration study. Arthritis Rheum 2006;54:1838–46.

14 Harris ST, Watts NB, Genant HK, et al. Effects of risedronate treatment on vertebral and nonvertebral fractures in women with postmenopausal osteoporosis: a randomized controlled trial. Vertebral Efficacy With Risedronate Therapy (VERT) Study Group. JAMA 1999;282:1344–52.

15 Reginster J, Minne HW, Sorensen OH, et al. Randomized trial of the effects of risedronate on vertebral fractures in women with established postmenopausal osteoporosis. Vertebral Efficacy with Risedronate Therapy (VERT) Study Group. Osteoporos Int 2000;11:83–91.

16 McClung MR, Geusens P, Miller PD, et al. Effect of risedronate on the risk of hip fracture in elderly women. Hip Intervention Program Study Group. N Engl J Med 2001;344:333–40.

17 Cranney A, Tugwell P, Adachi J, et al. Meta-analyses of therapies for postmenopausal osteoporosis. III. Meta-analysis of risedronate for the treatment of postmenopausa1 osteoporosis. Endocrine Rev 2002; 517–23.

18 UK Medicines Information Service. New medicines profile: zoledronic acid (Aclasta®) for osteoporosis. March 2008.

19 Woodis CB. Once-yearly administered intravenous zoledronic acid for postmenopausal osteoporosis. Ann Pharmacother. 2008;42(7):1085-9.

20 Black DM, Delmas PD, Eastell R, et al. Once-yearly zoledronic acid for treatment of postmenopausal osteoporosis. N Engl J Med 2007;356:1809–22.

21 Lyles KW, Colón-Emeric CS, Magaziner JS, Adachi JD, Pieper CF, Mautalen C, et al; for the HORIZON Recurrent Fracture Trial. Zoledronic Acid in Reducing Clinical Fracture and Mortality after Hip Fracture. N Engl J Med. 2007;357:nihpa40967.

22 McClung M, Recker R, Miller PD, et al. Intravenous zoledronic acid 5 mg in the treatment of postmenopausal women with low bone density previously treated with alendronate. Bone 2007;41:122–28.

23 Reid DM, Devogelaer JP, Saag K, et al. Zoledronic acid and risedronate in the prevention and treatment of glucocorticoid-induced osteoporosis (HORIZON): a multicentre, double-blind, double-dummy, randomised controlled trial. Lancet 2009;1253–63.

24 Compston J. Treatments for osteoporosis – looking beyond HORIZON. N Engl J Med 2007;356:1878–90.

25 Epstein S. Update of current therapeutic options for the treatment of postmenopausal osteoporosis. Clin Ther 2006;28:151–73.

26 Chaiamnuay S, Saag KG. Postmenopausal osteoporosis. What have we learned since the introduction of bisphosphonates? Rev Endocr Metab Disord 2006;7:101–12.

27 Cryer R, Bauer DC. Oral bisphosphonates and upper gastrointestinal tract problems: what is the evidence? Mayo Clin Proc 2002;77:1031–43.

28 Cramer JA, Silverman S. Persistence with bisphosphonate treatment for osteoporosis: finding the root of the problem. Am J Med 2006;119(suppl 1):S12–7.

29 Graham DY. What the gastroenterologist should know about the gastrointestinal safety profiles of bisphosphonates. Dig Dis Sci 2002;47:1665–78.

30 National Institute for Health and Clinical Excellence (NICE). Bisphosphonates (alendronate, etidronate, risedronate), selective oestrogen receptor modulators (raloxifene) and parathyroid hormone (teriparatide) for the secondary prevention of osteoporotic fragility fractures in postmenopausal women. Technology Appraisal 87 January 2005.

31 Reid IR. Osteonecrosis of the jaw: who gets it, and why? Bone 2009;4:44–10.

32 Bone HG, Hosking D, Devogelear JP, et al. Ten years' experience with alendronate for osteoporosis in postmenopausal women. N Engl J Med 2004;350:1189–99.

33 Sayed-Noor-AS, Sjoden-GO. Case reports: two femoral insufficiency fractures after long-term alendronate therapy. Clin Orthop Relat Res 2009;467;1921–6.

34 Somford MP, Draijer FW, Thomassen BJ, et al. Bilateral fractures of the femur diaphysis in a patient with rheumatoid arthritis on long-term treatment with alendronate: clues to the mechanism of increased bone fragility: J Bone Miner Res 2009;24:1736–40.

35 Abrahamsen B, Eiken P, Eastell R. Subtrochanteric and diaphyseal femur fractures in patients treated with alendronate: a register-based national cohort study. J Bone Miner Res 2009;24: 1095–102.

36 Abrahamsen B, Eiken P, Brixen K. Atrial fibrillation in fracture patients treated with oral bisphosphonates: J Intern Med 2009;265:581–92.

37 Grady D, Rubin SM, Petitti DB, et al. Hormone therapy to prevent disease and prolong life in postmenopausal women. Ann Intern Med 1992;117:1016–37.

38 Torgerson DJ, Bell-Syer SE. Hormone replacement therapy and prevention of nonvertebral fractures: a meta-analysis of randomized trials. JAMA 2001;285:2891–7.

39 Chlebowski RT, Hendrix SL, Langer RD, et al. Influence of estrogen plus progestin on breast cancer and mammography in healthy postmenopausal women: the Women's Health Initiative Randomized Trial. JAMA 2003;289:3243–53.

40 Beral V, Million Women Study Collaborators. Breast cancer and hormone-replacement therapy in the Million Women Study. Lancet. 2003;362:419–27.

41 Rapp SR, Espeland MA, Shumaker SA, et al. Effect of estrogen plus progestin on global cognitive function in postmenopausal women: the Women's Health Initiative Memory Study: a randomized controlled trial. JAMA 2003;289:2663–72.

42 Shumaker SA, Legault C, Rapp SR, et al. Estrogen plus progestin and the incidence of dementia and mild cognitive impairment in postmenopausal women: the Women's Health Initiative Memory Study: a randomized controlled trial. JAMA 2003;289:2651–62.

43 European Agency f or the Evaluation of Medicinal Products (EMEA). Public statement on recent publications regarding hormone therapy. London: The European Agency for the Evaluation of Medical Products; 3 December 2003.

44 Cauley JA, Robbins J, Chen Z, et al. Effects of estrogen plus progestin on risk of fracture and bone mineral density. The Women's Health Initiative Randomized Trial. JAMA 2003;290:1729–1738.

45 Ettinger B, Black DM, Mitlak BH, et al. Reduction of vertebral fracture risk in postmenopausal women with osteoporosis treated with raloxifene: results from a 3-year randomized clinical trial. JAMA 1999;282:637–645.

46 Lufkin EG, Whitaker MD, Nickelsen T, et al. Treatment of established postmenopausal osteoporosis with raloxifene: a randomized trial. J Bone Miner Res 1998;13:1747–54.

47 Martino S, Disch D, Dowsett SA, et al. Safety assessment of raloxifene over eight years in a clinical trial setting. Curr Med Res Opin 2005;21:1441–52.

48 Barrett - Conner E, Mosca L, Collins P et al. Effects of raloxifene on cardiovascular events and breast cancer in postmenopausal women. N Engl Med 2006;355:125–37.

49 Conbriza Summary of Product Characteristics. Available at: http://www.ema.europa.eu/docs/en_GB/document_library/EPAR_-_Product_Information/human/000913/WC500033577.pdf. Last accessed 19 August 2010.

50 Kanis JA, Johansson H, Oden A, McCloskey EV. Bazedoxifene reduces vertebral and clinical fractures in postmenopausal women at high risk assessed with FRAX®. Bone 2009;44:1049–54.

51 Miller PD, Chines AA, Christiansen C, et al. Effects of bazedoxifene on BMD and bone turnover in postmenopausal women: 2-yr results of a randomized, double-blind, placebo-, and active-controlled study. J Bone Miner Res 2008;23:525–35.

52 Silverman SL, Christiansen C, Genant HK, et al. Efficacy of bazedoxifene in reducing new vertebral fracture risk in postmenopausal women with osteoporosis: results from a 3-year, randomized, placebo-, and active-controlled clinical trial. J Bone Miner Res 2008;23:1923–34.

53 Overgaard K, Hansen MA, Jensen SB, et al. Effect of calcitonin given intranasally on bone mass and fracture rates in established osteoporosis: a dose response study. BMJ 1992;305:556–61.

54 Chesnut CH III, Silverman S, Andriano K, et al. A randomized trial of nasal spray salmon calcitonin in postmenopausal women with established osteoporosis: the Prevent Recurrence of Osteoporotic Fractures Study. PROOF study group. Am J Med 2000;109:267–76.

55 Deroisy R, Collette J, Albert A, et al. Comparison of the short-term effects of three oral calcium-vitamin D formulations and placebo on calcium metabolism. Curr Ther Res Clin Exp 1998;59:370–8.

56 Thomas JL, Meunier PJ. Evaluation of acceptability, tolerance and observance of a new calcium-vitamin D combination. Rhumatologie 1996;48:37–42.

57 Sheikh MS, Santa Ana CA, Nicar MJ, et al. Gastrointestinal absorption of calcium from milk and calcium salts. N Engl J Med 1987;317:532–6.

58 Trivedi DP, Doll R, Khaw KT. Effect of four monthly oral vitamin D_3 (cholecalciferol) supplementation on fractures and mortality in men and women living in the community: randomised double blind controlled trial. BMJ 2003;326:469–75.

59 Dempster DW, Cosman F, Kurland ES, et al. Effects of daily treatment with parathyroid hormone on bone microarchitecture and turnover in patients with osteoporosis: a paired biopsy study. J Bone Miner Res 2001;16:1846–53.

60 Neer RM, Arnaud CD, Zanchetta JR, et al. Effect of parathyroid hormone (1–34) on fractures and bone mineral density in postmenopausal women with osteoporosis. N Engl J Med 2001;344:1434–41.

61 Brixen KT, Christensen PM, Ejersted C, et al. Teriparatide (biosynthetic human parathyroid hormone 1–34): a new paradigm in the treatment of osteoporosis. Basic Clin Pharmacol Toxicol 2004;94:260–70.

62 Greenspan SL, Bone HG, Ettinger MP, et al. Effect of recombinant human parathyroid hormone (1–84) on vertebral fracture and bone mineral density in postmenopausal women with osteoporosis: a randomized trial. Ann Intern Med 2007 465:326–39.

63 Delmas PD. Treatment of postmenopausal osteoporosis. Lancet 2002;359:2018–26.

64 Marie PJ, Ammann P, Boivin G, et al. Mechanisms of action and therapeutic potential of strontium in bone. Calcif Tissue Int 2001;69:121–9.

65 Ammann P. Strontium ranelate: a novel mode of action leading to renewed bone quality. Osteoporos Int 2005;16(suppl 1):S11–5.

66 Meunier PJ, Roux C, Seeman E, et al. The effects of strontium ranelate on the risk of vertebral fracture in women with postmenopausal osteoporosis. N Engl J Med 2004;350:459–68.

67 Reginster JY, Meunier PJ. Strontium ranelate phase 2 dose-ranging studies: PREVOS and STRATOS studies. Osteoporos Int 2003;14(suppl 3):S56–65.

68 Blake GM, Fogelman I. Effect of bone strontium on BMD measurements. J Clin Densitom 2007;1:34–8.

69 Reginster JY, Seeman E, De Vernejoul MC, et al. Strontium ranelate reduces the risk of nonvertebral fractures in postmenopausal women with osteoporosis: Treatment of Peripheral Osteoporosis (TROPOS) study. J Clin Endocrinol Metab 2005;90:2816–22.

70 Hamdy NA. Denosumab: RANKL inhibition in the management of bone loss. Drugs Today 2008;44:7–21.

71 Bone HG, Bolognese MA, Yuen CK, et al. Effects of denosumab on bone mineral density and bone turnover in postmenopausal women. J Clin Endocrinol Metab 2008;93:2149–57.

72 Miller PD, Bolognese MA, Lewiecki EM, et al. Effect of denosumab on bone density and turnover in postmenopausal women with low bone mass after long-term continued, discontinued, and restarting of therapy: a randomized blinded phase 2 clinical trial. Bone 2008;43:22–9.

73 Cohen SB, Dore K, Lane NE, et al. Denosumab treatment effects on structural damage, bone mineral density, and bone turnover in rheumatoid arthritis. Arthritis Rheum 2008;58:1299–1309.

74 Cummings SR, San Martin J, McClung MR, et al. Denosumab for prevention of fractures in postmenopausal women with osteoporosis. N Engl J Med 2009;361:756–65.

75 McClung MR, Lewiecki EM, Cohen SB, et al. Denosumab in postmenopausal women with low bone mineral density. N Engl J Med 2006;354:821–31.

76 Lewiecki EM, Miller PD, McClung MR, et al. Two-year treatment with denosumab (AMG 162) in a randomized phase 2 study of postmenopausal women with low bone mineral density. J Bone Miner Res 2007;22:1832–41.

77 Brown-JP, Prince RL, Deal C, et al. Comparison of the effect of denosumab and alendronate on BMD and biochemical markers of bone turnover in postmenopausal women with low bone mass: a randomized, blinded, phase 3 trial. J Bone Miner Res 2009;24:153–61.

78 Scottish Intercollegiate Guidelines Network (SIGN). Management of osteoporosis: A national clinical guideline (No. 71), June 2003.

79 Cranney A, Guyatt G, Griffith L, et al. and the Osteoporosis Methodology Group and the Osteoporosis Research Advisory Group. Summary of meta-analyses of therapies for postmenopausal osteoporosis. Endocrine Rev 2002;23:570–578.

Chapter 8

Long-term management

Pain management

Pain is a universal result of acute fracture; furthermore, chronic pain is a common complication following hip and vertebral fracture and can have an adverse effect on patients' quality of life. Nevertheless, older patients are frequently undertreated for fracture pain, with a resultant increase in adverse outcomes [1]. For example, inadequate pain control after hip fracture is associated with poor short- and long-term functional recovery and a longer duration of hospitalization [2].

Acute pain relief

Acute fracture pain is best managed with opioids, ideally patient-controlled analgesia with morphine. Intravenous or oral opiates may be needed for subsequent pain control, particularly during physical therapy sessions. Yet clinicians are often reluctant to prescribe opioid medication to older adults, mainly due to concerns about precipitating or worsening delirium. A study of cognitively intact hip fracture patients found that although 40% reported severe or very severe pain, just 20% had a prescription for an analgesic agent. Patients with dementia fared even worse, receiving only one-third of the amount of opioids that cognitively intact patients received [3].

The fear that opioid medication might trigger delirium is not supported by the evidence. In the previously mentioned study, which followed 541 elderly patients with hip fracture, individuals receiving less than 10 mg/day of morphine sulphate were five times more likely to develop delirium after hip fracture than were patients who received more opiates. Furthermore, cognitively intact patients with severe pain had a 9-fold higher risk of developing delirium compared with those whose pain was adequately treated [3].

This study underscores the importance of aggressive pain control in older fracture patients, both to relieve suffering and to reduce the risk of delirium and its attendant complications.

Vertebral fracture

Acute vertebral fracture can cause almost intolerable pain for periods of weeks or months, especially in patients with several previous fractures [4]. The three forms of vertebral fracture – wedge, bioconcave and crush – are equally likely to produce pain. However the nature of pain may vary depending on the degree and severity of the fracture. The acute bone pain that occurs at the time of vertebral fracture normally resolves in 6–8 weeks. Management options in this setting include bracing, analgesics and functional restoration; open surgical management with decompression and stabilization is only rarely indicated [5].

Importantly, both prevalent and incident vertebral fractures can give rise to chronic back pain, with significant psychological and social consequences for the patient. Vertebral fractures can also lead to kyphosis and loss of height, both of which are associated with substantial levels of pain and disability [6]. Other complications of spinal deformity include increased energy expenditure, fatigue, decreased lung capacity and pulmonary function, poor mobility, and difficulties in the activities of daily living.

Kyphoplasty and vertebroplasty

Unlike most skeletal fractures, vertebral compression fractures have not traditionally been treated by attempts to stabilize the fracture and restore normal alignment and function. In the last decade, however, there has been considerable interest in two new minimally invasive procedures, kyphoplasty and vertebroplasty. Both techniques aim to stabilize the vertebral fracture, restore vertebral body height and relieve pain [5].

In vertebroplasty, a canula is inserted into the collapsed vertebral body and bone cement is injected. In kyphoplasty, balloon expansion of the vertebral body precedes cement injection. Evidence from case series and cohort studies suggests that both procedures offer immediate pain reduction as well as substantial functional improvement. Nevertheless the long-term efficacy and safety of vertebroplasty and kyphoplasty are unknown and the techniques have not been evaluated in randomized controlled trials. Surgical treatment therefore remains controversial and should be reserved for patients who fail to respond to non-surgical management options [1,5].

Exercise

Finally, exercise may be useful in controlling pain in patients with osteoporosis. In a prospective study of women with postmenopausal osteoporosis, those with the greatest improvement in aerobic fitness over a 4-year period reported a significantly greater reduction in pain than did women who were less fit [7]. In another study, women with osteoporosis were assessed periodically for levels of pain and activities of daily living. Those who participated in exercise sessions experienced a significant decrease in pain and an improvement in activities of daily living over the course of 6 months; in contrast, women in the control group had greater pain and decreased activity levels over the same period [8].

Compliance

Compliance and persistence with medication for osteoporosis is low, as is the case for other chronic diseases. The World Health Organization estimates that long-term adherence in chronic conditions averages only 50% [9]. It is likely to be even lower in disorders in which either the symptoms of the disease or the positive impact of treatment are not very evident to the patient.

Published rates of compliance with osteoporosis therapies vary widely but all studies show that it is suboptimal. One study found that 69% of patients prescribed raloxifene and 82% of patients given alendronate for osteoporosis remained compliant at 6-month follow-up [10]. In a separate study, 70.7% of patients who agreed to be treated with a bisphosphonate remained on therapy after 1 year [11]. More recently, a study using information about nearly 60,000 patients with osteoporosis found that 1-year compliance rates were less than 25% overall [12].

Impact of poor compliance

In patients with osteoporosis, the main consequence of poor compliance is a reduction in the antifracture efficacy of treatment. This in turn is associated with an increased risk of fracture, hospitalization, complications such as pain, nosocomial infection and pulmonary thromboembolism, and mortality. Thus, poor therapeutic compliance in osteoporosis is associated with suboptimal clinical outcomes, a decreased quality of life and increased healthcare costs.

Several studies have confirmed the link between medication compliance and antifracture efficacy. A 2-year study of more than 11,000 women with osteoporosis found that the risk of fracture was 16% lower in those who took ≥80% of their prescribed medication than in less compliant patients (Figure 8.1) [13]. Another study found a 26% difference in fracture risk between compliant and non-compliant patients [14]. In a large registry study, compliance with medication over a 1-year period reduced the risk of hip and vertebral fracture by 62% and 40%, respectively, compared with non-compliance [15].

Unsurprisingly, compliance with bisphosphonate therapy is also correlated with changes in bone mineral density (BMD) and biomarkers of bone resorption. In a study of patients receiving glucocorticoids, BMD was maintained in individuals who were compliant with bisphosphonate

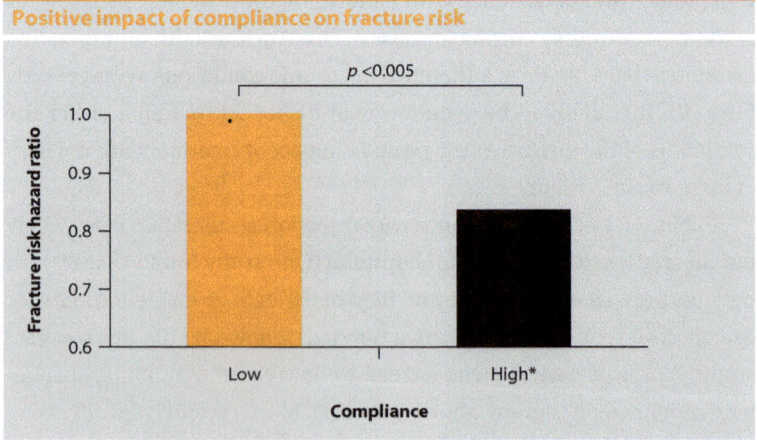

Positive impact of compliance on fracture risk

Figure 8.1 Positive impact of compliance on fracture risk. High = drug available to cover ≥ 80% of the time. High compliance group had 16% reduction in fracture rate. Data from Caro et al [13].

therapy; in contrast, those who discontinued bisphosphonates early but continued on glucocorticoids experienced substantial loss of BMD at the spine and hip (Figure 8.2) [15].

Reasons for poor compliance

Many factors influence long-term compliance and persistence with osteoporosis medication. As noted above, osteoporosis does not necessarily produce symptoms. Without obvious evidence of disease, patients may not believe their diagnosis or perceive that they are suffering from a severe condition. Furthermore, measures of therapeutic outcome, such as increases in BMD or reductions in biomarkers of bone turnover, are not readily available. Patients are therefore unable to monitor their response to medication and gain feedback regarding the benefits.

A recent survey of 502 women with postmenopausal osteoporosis offers important insights into the reasons for non-compliance [16]. All women had been prescribed a bisphosphonate for osteoporosis, yet over one-third had discontinued treatment. Furthermore, over half of the women in the survey had experienced drawbacks with their treatment, even if they were still compliant. The most frequently cited reasons for

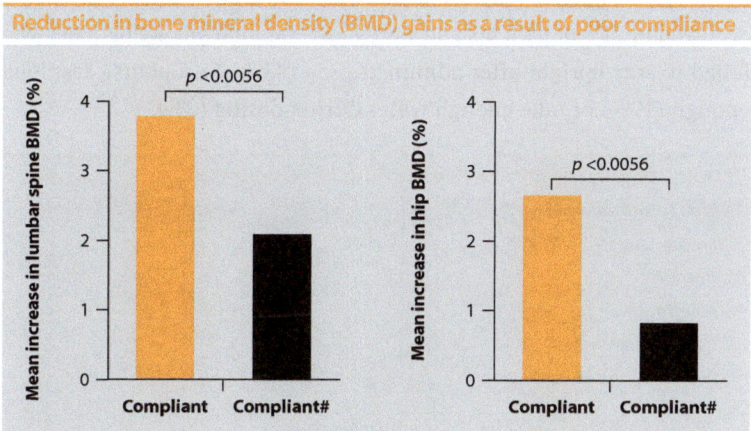

Figure 8.2 Reduction in bone mineral density (BMD) gains as a result of poor compliance. 176 previously untreated women with postmenopausal osteoporosis, receiving oestrogen or bisphoshonates. Compliant defined as those achieving ≥ 66% compliance. Non-compliant defined as those achieving < 66% compliance; compliance = number of months of drug therapy. Data from Yood et al. [11].

non-compliance were the stringent dosing schedule, adverse events, not feeling that treatment had worked, or not believing that the disease that needed treating (Figure 8.3).

Several studies have shown that patients find the strict dosing instructions for bisphosphonates difficult to follow. Fasting (overnight for at least 6 hours prior to taking the medication and 30–60 minutes after administration) and posture requirements (staying upright for 30–60 minutes after taking the medication) can be inconvenient and often not feasible in the daily routine. These restrictions interfere not only with eating and drinking but also with taking other medications, especially if they need to be taken with food.

Gastrointestinal side effects are another reason for non-compliance with bisphosphonates and occur more often in the community than was reported in the pivotal clinical trials (see Chapter 7 for a detailed discussion of the tolerability of bisphosphonates). Importantly, failure to adhere strictly to dosing instructions increases the risk of oesophageal side effects and reduces drug absorption [17].

In a study of 219 women receiving alendronate for the treatment of osteoporosis, 26% did not follow dosing instructions despite receiving counselling and written instructions [18]. Upper GI adverse events occurred in 21% of patients and were most common among patients who failed to stay upright after administration (43% of dropouts), fast long enough (19%) or take enough water during dosing (3%).

Reasons for non-compliance with bisphosphonate therapy for osteoporosis	
Reason for non-compliance	**Percentage (n=275)**
Dislike any long-term medication	5
Frequency	9
Inconvenience	10
Don't feel this medication works	11
Remembering to take medication	12
Fasting	17
Side effects	20
Staying upright	23

Figure 8.3 Reasons for non-compliance with bisphosphonate therapy for osteoporosis.
Note: some women stated ≥ 1 reason. Data from International Osteoporosis Foundation [16].

Methods for improving tolerability and compliance

Experience with oral bisphosphonates suggests that a proven efficacy and tolerability profile is not enough to ensure high compliance with osteoporosis treatment. Alternative strategies that have shown promise in improving compliance include less-frequent dosing regimens and patient education initiatives.

Extending the dosing interval to improve compliance

Less-frequent dosing reduces disruption to patients' daily lives and appears to significantly improve compliance and persistence with therapy without loss of antifracture efficacy. Both alendronate and risedronate are licensed for weekly dosing and, as well as having the convenience of taking only one tablet per week, are widely accepted to be at least as effective as daily regimens. The comparable efficacies of daily and weekly regimens of these drugs has been inferred from equivalent increases in BMD (a validated surrogate marker for antifracture efficacy) and decreases in bone turnover markers (Figure 8.4) [19,20].

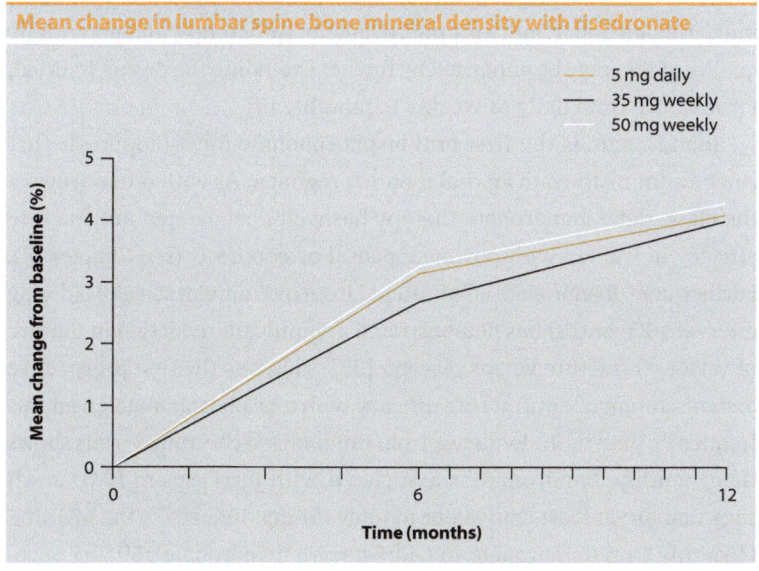

Figure 8.4 Mean change in lumbar spine bone mineral density with risedronate. Mean change in bone mineral density of the lumbar spine with risedronate. Data from Brown et al. [20].

In randomized clinical trials of oral bisphosphonates, patients have consistently expressed a preference for weekly versus daily dosing [21,22]. Weekly regimens are considered by patients to be more convenient than daily regimens and most likely to allow them to achieve long-term adherence to treatment [23,24].

The clear patient preference for less frequent dosing has been shown to translate into improved adherence with therapy, although it remains suboptimal. An analysis of administrative claims data on 2741 women with postmenopausal osteoporosis found that patients prescribed a daily bisphosphonate discontinued treatment after 185 days, on average, compared with 227 days for those prescribed weekly therapy [24]. After 12 months of therapy, 44.2% versus 31.7% of women prescribed weekly versus daily bisphosphonates, respectively, had persisted with treatment (Figure 8.5).

Analyses of other healthcare databases indicate that 1-year persistence is increased by 12–29% among patients given weekly bisphosphonate rather than daily dosing regimens. Nevertheless, less than half of patients receiving a weekly regimen persist with therapy for 12 months, indicating an opportunity for improvement. Adherence, and potentially quality of life, may be enhanced by further extending the dosing interval, for instance from daily or weekly to monthly [9].

Ibandronate is the first oral bisphosphonate for osteoporosis that can be administered in an oral monthly regimen. As with other drugs in the class, daily ibandronate therapy has well-documented antifracture efficacy in women with postmenopausal osteoporosis (see Chapter 7). Furthermore, ibandronate administered in an intermittent schedule (dosing interval >2 months) has demonstrated a significant reduction in the risk of vertebral fracture versus placebo [25]. This was the first prospective demonstration of antifracture efficacy with a bisphosphonate given less frequently than daily. Evidence from randomized controlled trials shows that monthly ibandronate is associated with increases in BMD at all sites that are at least equivalent to daily dosing. Indeed, in the MOBILE (Monthly Oral iBandronate In LadiEs) trial, ibandronate 150 mg once-monthly was superior to the daily regimen in terms of change in lumbar spine BMD and markers of bone turnover (Figure 8.6) [26]. Importantly, monthly treatment showed a good tolerability profile, with an incidence of adverse effects similar to that of the daily regimen [25].

Women with postmenopausal osteoporosis have expressed a strong preference for monthly versus weekly oral bisphosphonate therapy in randomized clinical trials. The BALTO I and II (Boniva ALendronate

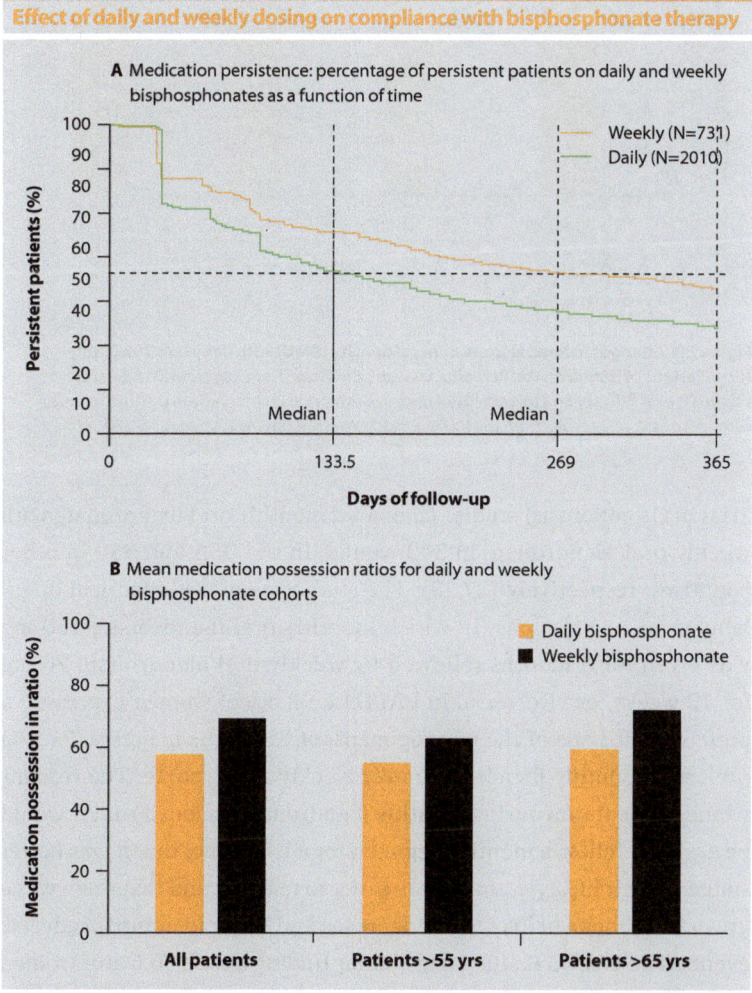

Figure 8.5 Effect of daily and weekly dosing on compliance with bisphosphonate therapy.
Reproduced with permission from Cramer JA, Silverman S. Persistence with bisphosphonate treatment for osteoporosis: finding the root of the problem. Am J Med 2006;119(suppl 1):S12–7.

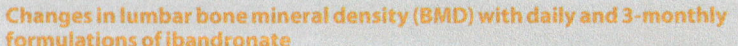

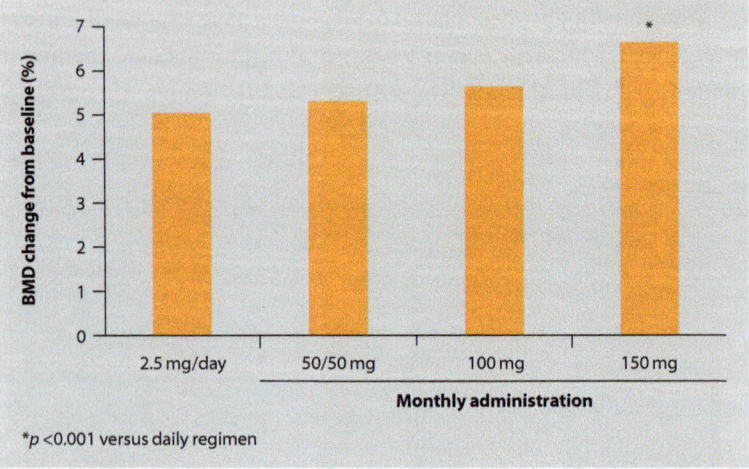

*p <0.001 versus daily regimen

Figure 8.6 Changes in lumbar bone mineral density (BMD) with daily and 3-monthly formulations of ibandronate. Reproduced with permission from Reginster JY, Adami S, Lakatos P, et al. Efficacy and tolerability of once-monthly oral ibandronate in postmenopausal osteoporosis: 2 year results from the MOBILE study. Ann Rheum Dis 2006A;65:654–61.

Trial in Osteoporosis) studies compared monthly oral ibandronate with weekly oral alendronate in 342 women in the USA and 350 in other countries, respectively [27,28]. The studies employed identical open-label crossover designs, in which monthly oral ibandronate 150 mg was given for 3 months followed by weekly oral alendronate 70 mg for 12 weeks, or vice versa. In BALTO I, 92.6% of women expressed a preference for one of the two regimens, of which the majority (71.4%) preferred monthly ibandronate over weekly alendronate. The reasons women gave for favouring monthly ibandronate included that it would be easier to follow a monthly regimen for a long time; that it was better suited to their lifestyle; that it was easier to tolerate; and that there was a greater likelihood of long-term adherence and better tolerance of adverse events. The BALTO II study had similar findings, with 76.6% of women who expressed an opinion preferring monthly ibandronate (Figure 8.7). Again, the reasons cited were its greater convenience, ease of long-term adherence and better fit to lifestyle.

The hypothesis that patient preference for a medication encourages compliance has recently been addressed in a British study, PERSIST [30]. Patients were randomized to treatment with monthly ibandronate (plus a patient support programme; n = 547) or to weekly alendronate (n = 529). Patient support was offered only to ibandronate-treated patients, to reflect current UK standard practice. At 6-month follow-up, persistence with treatment was 47% greater in the ibandronate group than in the alendronate group: the number of patients discontinuing treatment was 107 in the ibandronate group (20%) and 134 in the alendronate group (25%) (p = 0.023). This is in line with the reported 12–29% relative improvements in 1-year persistence with weekly versus daily dosing [9]. Secondary endpoints, such as the proportion of patients remaining on treatment at study end and proportion of patients discontinuing from the study, also favoured the monthly regimen.

Educating patients about the long-term treatment plan

Patient education is used in the management of many diseases as a method for improving compliance. It is particularly beneficial in chronic

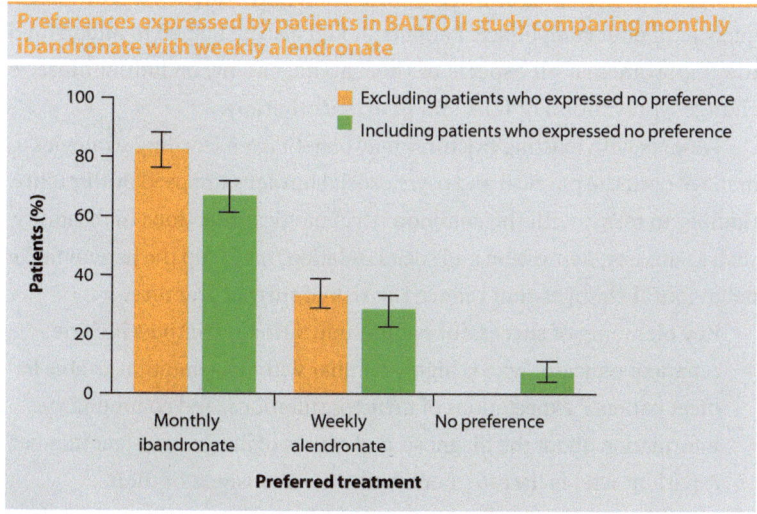

Figure 8.7 Preferences expressed by patients in BALTO II study comparing monthly ibandronate with weekly alendronate. 95% confidence intervals are shown. For patients expressing a preference, p < 0.0001 for difference between monthly ibandronate and weekly alendronate groups. Data from Hadji et al. [29].

conditions that can be asymptomatic for long periods before a serious event occurs. Many primary care providers have established enduring, trusting relationships with their patients; this bond promotes good communication and patient confidence in the recommendations made for their care. Primary carers may therefore be ideally placed to convince patients to persist with medication and to monitor them over time to identify issues that might affect compliance.

To improve the likelihood of good outcome in a patient with osteoporosis, the clinician should focus on providing information about the disease state and the consequences of non-compliance. For treatments with strict dosing requirements such as bisphosphonates, patients should be educated about the reasons for the administration guidelines – i.e. that they ensure that the drug is absorbed properly and reduce the likelihood of side effects.

Other goals of education include increasing patients' knowledge about the condition and clarifying misconceptions. This should include information about diagnosis, risk factors, complications, treatments and prognosis. For patients who have not yet sustained a fracture, it is important to highlight the urgent need for treatment and the consequences of poor compliance. Patients should also be helped to understand the importance of all aspects of their management, including lifestyle changes, prevention of falls and pharmacotherapy.

Patients with existing fractures may benefit from learning strategies to manage both the physical and psychosocial burdens imposed by disability. Coming to terms with the common psychological reactions to disability, such as anxiety, depression and social isolation, may help the patient make behavioural changes that reduce the risk of further fracture.

Key elements of successful patient education initiatives include:
- A patient educator who is highly familiar with the condition, is able to meet patients' expectations of their consultations, and communicates information about the diagnosis and causes of illness in a clear manner.
- A patient who is literate, perceives the seriousness of their condition and believes that treatment is effective and worthwhile.
- A healthcare setting that is unthreatening, such as community-based support groups.

Patient education has been demonstrated to improve medication compliance and persistence across broad range of conditions, although few studies have focused on patients with osteoporosis. One study assessed a multifactorial intervention in 58 patients with a forearm fracture [31]. Each patient received: educational materials on osteoporosis, recommended calcium intake and recurrent facture risk; an appointment for bone densitometry testing; and a consultation with a primary care physician. The rate of successful intervention was 45% among study participants versus 16% in the general population. Women who were already being treated for osteoporosis at the time of fracture were much more likely to remain on treatment for 6 months compared with those who were newly started on therapy. In addition, 67% of women with T-scores ≤1.5 were compliant with treatment at 6-month follow-up, compared with 100% of those with borderline or normal T-scores. These data highlight the need for enhanced education initiatives among patients newly diagnosed with osteoporosis.

Self-management is another approach to improving outcomes and emphasizes the central role of the patient in managing his or her own illness. Better Choices for Bone Health is a recently developed community-based programme that aims to motivate patients to comply with long-term behaviours that improve bone health [32]. It consists of five 2- to 3-hour sessions that are co-chaired by a healthcare professional and a patient with osteoporosis. During the sessions participants engage in both individual and group work, including lectures and discussions. A description of the session contents is given in Figure 8.8

References

1   Colón-Emeric CS, Saag KG. Osteoporotic fractures in older adults. Best Pract Res Clin Rheumatol 2006;20:695–706.
2   Morrison RS, Magaziner J, McLaughlin MA, et al. The impact of post-operative pain on outcomes following hip fracture. Pain 2003;103:303–11.
3   Morrison RS, Magaziner J, Gilbert M, et al. Relationship between pain and opioid analgesics on the development of delirium following hip fracture. J Gerontol A Biol Sci Med Sci 2003;58:76–81.
4   Ismail AA, Cooper C, Felsenberg D, et al. Number and type of vertebral deformities: epidemiological characteristics and relation to back pain and height loss. Osteoporos Int 1999;9:206–13.
5   Kim DH, Vaccaro AR. Osteoporotic compression fractures of the spine; current options and considerations for treatment. Spine J. 2006 Sep–Oct;6:479–87.
6   Silverman SL. Quality of life issues in osteoporosis. Curr Rheumatol Rep 2005;7:39–45.

Session contents in 'Choices for Better Bone Health', a community-based management programme	
Key learning points	**Bone health behaviours**
Session 1: It's never too late	
• Osteoporosis is not an inevitable part of aging • It's never too early and never too late to improve your bone health • You can make your bones healthier	Getting enough calcium and vitamin D is an important first step in making bones healthier
Session 2 : There's more you can do	
• You have choices of osteporosis medicines that can help make you bones healthier • You and your healthcare professional can select the right osteoporosis medicine for you • No one medicine is right for everyone	You can take your osteoporosis medicine as recommended by your healthcare professional
Session 3: Taking charge	
• Osteoporosis may lead to changes in your social roles • Osteoporosis may cause negative feelings and thoughts • A healthy outlook about your osteoprosis can lead to changes in those negative feelings	You can manage the chronic pain and discomfort of osteoporosis
Session 4: Living safe and sound	
• You can change your environment to make it safer and prevent falls • You can perform your daily activities in ways that reduce your risk of fracture	You can do exercise that should reduce your risk of falling and fractures
Session 5: Putting it all together	
• Your body changes with osteoporosis • You can be stylish with osteoporosis	You can develop a personal plan for better bone health

Figure 8.8 Session contents in 'Choices for Better Bone Health', a community-based management programme. Adapted with permission from Gold DT, Silverman SL. Osteoporosis self-management: choices for better bone health. South Med J 2004;97:551–4.

7 Harrison JE, Chow R, Dornan J, et al. Evaluation of a program for rehabilitation of osteoporotic patients (PRO): 4-year follow-up. Osteoporos Int 1993;3:13–7.

8 Helmes E, I-lodsmiiani A, Iazowski D, ct al. A questionnaire to evaluate disability in osteoporotic patients with vertebral compression fractures. J Gerontol A Biol Sci 1990;50:M191–8.

9 Reginster JY, Rabenda V. Patient preference in the management of postmenopausal osteoporosis with bisphosphonates. Clin Intervent Aging 2006;1:415–423.

10 Segal E, Tamir A, Ish-Shalom S. Compliance of osteoporotic patients with different treatment regimens. Isr Med Assoc J 2003;5:859–62.

11 Yood RA, Emani S, Reed JI, Lewis BE, et al. Compliance with pharmacologic therapy for osteoporosis. Osteoporos Int 2003;14:965–968.

12 McCombs JS, Thiebaud P, McLaughlin-Miley C, et al. Compliance with drug therapies for the treatment and prevention of osteoporosis. Maturitas 2004;48:271–87.

13 Caro JJ, Ishak KJ, Huybrechts KF, et al. The impact of compliance with osteoporosis therapy on fracture rates in actual practice. Osteoporos Int 2004;15:1003–1008.

14 Siris E, Rosen CJ, Harris ST, et al. Adherence to bisphosphonate therapy: relationship to bone fractures at 24 months in women with post-menopausal osteoporosis. Presented at the

National Osteoporosis Foundation 6th International Symposium on Osteoporosis; April 6–9, 2005; Washington, DC.

15 Emkey R, Delmas PD, Goemaere S, et al. Changes in bone mineral density following discontinuation or continuation of alendronate therapy in glucocorticoid-treated patients: a retrospective, observational study. Arthritis Rheum 2003;48:1102–8.

16 International Osteoporosis Foundation (IOF). The adherence gap: why osteoporosis patients don't continue with treatment. A European report highlighting the gap between the beliefs of people with osteoporosis and the perceptions of their physicians. Nyon: IOF, 2005.

17 Cramer JA, Silverman S. Persistence with bisphosphonate treatment for osteoporosis: finding the root of the problem. Am J Med 2006;119(suppl 1):S12–7.

18 Hamilton B, McCoy K, Taggart H. Tolerability and compliance with risedronate in clinical practice. Osteoporos Int 2003;14:259–62.

19 Schnitzer T, Bone HG, Crepaldi G, et al. Therapeutic equivalence of alendronate 70 mg once-weekly and alendronate 10 mg daily in the treatment of osteoporosis. Alendronate Once-Weekly Study Group. Aging 2000;12:1–12.

20 Brown JP, Kendler DL, McClung MR, et al. The efficacy and tolerability of risedronate once a week for the treatment of postmenopausal osteoporosis. Calcif Tissue Int. 2002;71:103–111.

21 Simon JA, Lewiecki EM, Smith ME, et al. Patient preference for once-weekly alendronate 70 mg versus once-daily alendronate 10 mg: a multicenter, randomized, open-label, crossover study. Clin Ther 2002;24:1871–86.

22 Kendler D, Kung AW, Fuleihan Gel-H, et al. Patients with osteoporosis prefer once weekly to once daily dosing with alendronate. Maturitas 2004;48:243–51.

23 Recker RR, Gallagher R, MacCosbe PE. Effect of dosing frequency on bisphosphonate medication adherence in a large longitudinal cohort of women. Mayo Clin Proc 2005;80:856–61.

24 Cramer JA, Amonkar MM, Hebborn A, et al. Compliance and persistence with bisphosphonate dosing regimens among women with postmenopausal osteoporosis. Curr Med Res Opin 2005;21:1453–60.

25 Chesnut III CH, Skag A, Christiansen C, et al. Effects of oral ibandronate administered daily or intermittently on fracture risk in postmenopausal osteoporosis. J Bone Miner Res 2004;19:1241–9.

26 Reginster JY, Adami S, Lakatos P, et al. Efficacy and tolerability of once-monthly oral ibandronate in postmenopausal osteoporosis: 2 year results from the MOBILE study. Ann Rheum Dis 2006;65:654–61.

27 Emkey R, Koltun W, Beusterien K, et al. Patient preference for once-monthly ibandronate versus once-weekly alendronate in a randomized, open-label, cross-over trial: the Boniva Alendronate Trial in Osteoporosis (BALTO). Curr Med Res Opin 2005;21:1895–903.

28 Hadji P, Benhamou C-L, Devas V, Masanauskaite D, Barrett-Connor E. Women with postmenopausal osteoporosis prefer once-monthly oral ibandronate to weekly oral alendronate: results of BALTO II. Abstract presented at 6th European Congress on Clinical and Economic Aspects of Osteoporosis and Osteoarthritis, Vienna, Austria, 15–18 March 2006.

29 Hadji P, Minne H, Pfeifer M, et al. Treatment preference for monthly oral ibandronate and weekly oral alendronate in women with postmenopausal osteoporosis: a randomized, crossover study (BALTO II). Joint Bone Spine. 2008; 75:303–10.

30 Cooper A, Drake J, Brankin E, et al. Treatment persistence with once-monthly ibandronate and patient support vs. once-weekly alendronate: results from the PERSIST study. Int J Clin Pract 2006;60:896–905.

31 Cuddihy MT, Amadio PC, Gabriel SE, et al. A prospective clinical practise intervention to improve osteoporosis management following distal forearm fracture. Osteoporosis Int 2004;15:695–700.

32 Gold DT, Silverman SL. Osteoporosis self-management: choices for better bone health. South Med J 2004;97:551–4.